MANAGING YOUR BUSINESS

BUSINESS

MILADY'S GUIDE
TO THE SALON

MANAGING YOUR BUSINESS

MILADY'S GUIDE TO THE SALON

LESLIE EDGERTON

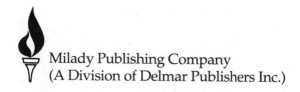
Milady Publishing Company
(A Division of Delmar Publishers Inc.)

NOTICE TO THE READER

Publisher: Catherine Frangie
Developmental Editor: Joseph Miranda
Senior Project Editor: Laura Gulotty
Freelance Project Editor: Pamela Fuller
Production Manager: John Mickelbank
Art Design/Supervisor: Susan Mathews

Delmar Publishers' Online Services

To access Delmar on the World Wide Web, point your browser to:
http://www.delmar.com/delmar.html
To access through Gopher: gopher://gopher.delmar.com
(Delmar Online is part of "thomson.com", an Internet site with information on more than 30 publishers of the International Thomson Publishing organization.)
For information on our products and services:
email: info@delmar.com
or call 800-347-7707

Copyright ©1994
Milady Publishing Company
(A Division of Delmar Publishers Inc.)

For information address:
Milady Publishing Company
(A Division of Delmar Publishers Inc.)
3 Columbia Circle, Box 12519
Albany, NY 12212-2519

Printed in the United States of America
Published simultaneously in Canada
by Nelson Canada
a division of the Thomson Corporation.

3 4 5 6 7 8 9 10 XXX 00 99 98 97

Library of Congress Cataloging-in-Publication Data

Edgerton, Leslie.
    Managing your business: Milady's guide to the salon/Leslie
Edgerton.
        p.   cm.
    Includes index.
    ISBN 1-56253-084-4
    1. Beauty shops—Management.   I. Title.
TT965.E32   1994
646.7'2'068—dc20   93-8191
                                                                       CIP

CONTENTS

ACKNOWLEDGEMENTS

An author of a book is very lucky. He or she gets to have his or her name prominently displayed as the creator of a work, when in actuality, any book, especially one such as this, is the product of many minds and hands. I owe a large debt to Catherine Frangie, my editor, who had the foresight to see the need in our industry for a book on this topic and the faith that I could deliver a quality product (not to mention the long-suffering patience that kept her smiling through my requests for "just one more extension, *pleeeeeze, Cathy!*" that I put her through!). Large doses of gratitude must go as well to such contributors as my talented photographer Matt Newbauer, who did a thoroughly professional job with not very much time in which to perform his miracles; JeriSue Petrie who let me steal (and graciously use) large chunks of her small business lore and expertise; and those helpful individuals such as my talented bean-counter and financial advisor Glen Allie; our friendly and helpful banker Maureen Rehmer for all her financial tips; and Ron Mataya of Nuco (Leprechaun Salon Software) for his insights into salon computer systems. This book would still be only half done if it were not for my two wondrous computer gurus who got me up and running—many thanks to JoAnne Soest, who took me by the hand and showed me computers could be easy to learn, and to Bob Masbaum, who invested his genius and time into getting my "gray boxes" up and running and without whom I would still be staring at components and scratching my head!

Thanks to all the others who helped along the way, and an especial round of kudos to my wife, Mary, who took on many of my other jobs so I could prepare this book, and to Cindy McQueen, our Salon Coordinator who contributed in a thousand and one ways as well.

DEDICATION

My life, I feel, has been singularly blessed with riches, and the riches I speak of are not material in composition but spiritual and are derived chiefly from my family. It is to my family, therefore, that I dedicate this book, as I hope I dedicate most substantive elements of life; chiefly, to my beautiful wife and partner, Mary, and the three greatest kids in the world, Britney, Sienna, and Mikey-Bud. A dedication is a highly personal glimpse at the inner workings of a person's heart and affords the writer an opportunity to give testimonial to those he truly respects, and it is with this spirit that I also dedicate this book to my late father, Leslie "Bud" Edgerton, who taught me that a job worth doing is worth doing right.

INTRODUCTION

Many more years ago than I would care to admit to, I opened my first hairstyling salon. Looking back on that experience today, I am amazed that I was able to keep food on the table for my family considering the way I ran that business. Fortunately for me (and my dependents!) times were such that haircutters made money in spite of all the business mistakes we committed. Today's economic climate affords no such luxuries. No longer can we manage "by the seat of our pants" as we used to. The marketplace is too fierce to allow it.

I'd like to think I did some things right as well—enough to survive—and I hope I've recognized those elements that were done properly and retained them. The savviest business technique I ever employed was to provide the best quality service I was capable of and charge a fair price for it. That is probably what kept me in business then, and I think I will always use that premise as the cornerstone of any salon I ever own.

Unfortunately, in today's world that just isn't enough. It's a good start, granted, and shows a strong sense of ethics and morality which are important qualities, but the naked truth is that good intentions; hard, honest labor; and forthrightness are simply not sufficient any longer.

Did you know that bankers or venture capitalists looking for places to invest their money would rather put their resources into a good management team with an average to even mediocre product or service than into an excellent product or service with an average or mediocre management team? They know that good management is much more important than the product or service, at least as far as returning a profit and running a successful business are concerned. It would be a nice world if we were rewarded by the quality of our haircuts, but the hard truth is that we will be rewarded more for an average haircut marketed by outstanding management and marketing. Now, if you can put superior management behind an outstanding product or service, then you've got the best possible combination.

The purpose of this book is to provide you with a blueprint for opening and running a successful salon. Without such a blueprint, it becomes exceedingly difficult to compete with those salons that are on the right track. If you are still of the mind that a great product (i.e., your fantastic haircutting ability) is all you need, look around at some of the salons in your own town that have been in business a long time and are always busy. I'll bet a chunk of change that many, if not most, of the owners of those salons aren't necessarily the best haircutters in town. They may *employ* the best hair designers—chances are pretty good that they do—but they themselves may not be that gifted in the art of haircutting and design. It is important to have good skills, but it is *even more important* to have good management skills and techniques. If you don't believe me, ask that banker you know who drives a new car every year and wears Sulka ties which *he'd* rather back with his money—the best widget in town or the best business manager with the worst widget!

Those are the cold, harsh facts of reality. I won't sugar-coat what is in store for you out there when you open a salon. It's tough, my friend. There is hope, however, as well as grounds for a great deal of optimism for your new venture. There are proven ways to succeed, time-tested methods of business that work, over and over. *Managing Your Business: Milady's Guide to the Salon* will show you those methods—show you how to open a new salon and run it at a profit.

When I opened my first salon in the late sixties, there were no such texts. Most salon owners at that time were lucky to have completed high school, let alone any advanced business or college courses. Even today, though many more of us have attained higher levels of education, up until now there has been a dearth of books directed specifically toward salon entrepreneurs, and though some general business tactics may have been learned, large parts of the salon business picture were usually missing. *Managing Your Business* provides a complete picture that anyone, from the first-time salon owner to the owner of a national chain of salons, will find instructive and motivating, and an effective map to success.

As we inch closer to the twenty-first century, the world becomes an increasingly complex place in which to live. The attainment and utilization of knowledge are our only sure means of survival. Treat the book you have in your hand as a primary weapon in your arsenal, but don't stop there. Read every bit of material you can get your hands on. It truly is a jungle out there, but the salon owner who possesses the right knowledge and information will be the survivor, and even more importantly, the *prosperous* survivor. In the introduction to my last book on stylist-client communication, *You and Your Client: Milady's Human Relations for Cosmetology,* I made the statement that "twenty percent of the salons do eighty percent of the business." That statement is just as true today, if not more so. The tools that will enable you to be included in that affluent twenty-percent group are readily available if you know where to look—you hold one of them in your hand right now.

Let's begin what should be the adventure of our lives—owning a business!

ABOUT THE AUTHOR

Salon owner Leslie Edgerton is a sixteen-time winner of state hairstyling championships and trophies in Indiana, Illinois, and Michigan. A successful hairstylist and designer for twenty-five years, Edgerton has also been a platform artist for Clairol. He is a contributing editor to *Hair and Beauty News;* has written numerous articles for such publications as *Brides, Bridal Trends,* and *National Beauty School Journal;* and had technicals and photos of his work in such magazines as *Touts, Dixie Magazine,* and *Gambit.* He was a contributing author to Milady's *Standard Textbook of Cosmetology* and is the author of *You and Your Clients: Milady's Human Relations for Cosmetology.*

Edgerton has also been featured on the television show "PM Magazine" and on Cox Cable in an in-depth interview with Paul Cimino. A graduate of Indiana University, he is presently taking graduate courses toward an MFA in writing. Along with nonfiction, Edgerton also writes novels and short fiction. He has had many short stories published in literary magazines and anthologies and won a national award for his novel *Spatterdashers.* He and his wife, Mary, own and operate Bold Strokes Hair Designers in Ft. Wayne, Indiana.

C H A P T E R
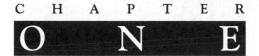

Congratulations! You have decided to open your own business, or so I assume, by the very act of purchasing a copy of this book. Or perhaps you already have an established salon and are looking for ways to improve it. Again, congratulations—by seeking additional knowledge you manifest the kind of spirit and planning necessary to achieve success and set yourself apart from the rest of the pack.

As you are doubtless aware, only one in three businesses are still around five years after starting up. Only by proper planning can anyone hope to be one of the survivors, and proper planning can not only help ensure your salon's survival, but make it a solid success. (Figure 1.1)

Many fallacies abound concerning owning your own business. It is best to be aware of those misconceptions so as not to fall victim to them and end up with a failed effort. For instance, if you think you can start up on a shoestring and wing it, please dissuade yourself of that notion. Undercapitalization is a major cause of business failures. Most new salons don't begin to earn a profit for at least a year.

Another myth is the thought that "I'll be my own boss." Well, yes, you *can* be, provided you don't have to deal with clients, salespersons, or investors. If any of those people are crucial to your success, then you really aren't your own boss.

Yet another misconception is that you'll be rich instantly. Wrong again! Most salons, no matter how busy, will still require your energy, time, and talent to manage growth and create wealth.

FIGURE 1.1
Congratulations on your grand opening! Proper planning will ensure that your new salon will be a solid success.

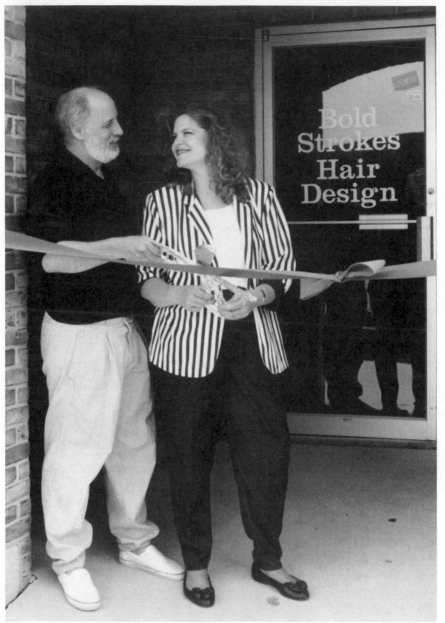

Rid yourself of all the misconceptions you may have about owning your own business. It will take hard work and good planning to have a realistic chance of succeeding, but if you plan well and are willing to work hard you do have a good chance of making it.

STRUCTURING YOUR BUSINESS

The first step in planning for your salon is to determine how it will be set up. Your accountant and lawyer can give you the best advice here. There are three basic ways to structure a salon.

The easiest system (not necessarily the best) is a sole proprietorship or partnership. Legally, neither requires that anything be set up in writing, but a partnership agreement is recommended as a safeguard if that is the form you choose. A proprietorship is held personally responsible for taxes and liabilities of the salon. Taxes on income of $60,000 a year or more are generally higher for a sole proprietor (at the time of this writing) and partnerships, and their income is reported on individual tax forms.

A limited partnership may be formed to limit the liability of one or more partners and to define the role and liabilities of a partner who is usually only an investor and has no management responsibilities. This agreement must usually be filed with the secretary of state in most states.

A corporation exists apart from the people who create it, becoming a legal entity unto itself. In general, corporations, especially S-corporation elections, are favorable ways of conducting business when taxable income reaches $60,000 a year or more. Personal liabilities are fewer as well.

What is the best way for you to do business? The best source of advice on this is probably your attorney and/or accountant.

TYPES OF SALONS

The National Cosmetology Association (NCA) identifies three basic types of salons: the **specialty salon,** providing specific services; the **full-service salon,** providing all services; and the **service and retail combination salon,** providing services and a line of retail goods. You must choose which of those kinds of salons best fits you and your own goals. The NCA has brochures and other material available to the new salon owner. They are listed in Appendix A, along with many other valuable resources.

NEW VERSUS ESTABLISHED SALONS

If it is to be a new salon, you will want to resolve some other questions. Do you plan on opening an entirely new enterprise or purchasing an existing salon, or are you investigating franchise systems? Each has its pluses and minuses, but whichever you are considering, you will want to be aware of certain things.

For instance, if you are thinking of purchasing a franchise, are you first of all happy with the image the franchise projects? Remember, the reputation of the franchise will become yours. If what you have in mind is a haute couture kind of salon, would you be happy in a budget operation, no matter how much income it brought in? Other questions about franchises you should seek answers to are:

- What capital is required?
- What are franchise fees and payments or royalties?
- What are the certified profits of other franchises in the franchise system?
- What is the franchise track record?
- How dependent or independent will you be allowed to be?
- How can you terminate the agreement?
- Can you sell the franchise and under what terms?
- Do your abilities match up well with those of other franchisees?
- What services are offered?
- Are any elements of the franchise agreement illegal in your state?
- Has your lawyer reviewed everything, and what is his or her advice?

Purchasing an already-established salon may or may not be a good idea. Again, there are areas you should investigate and questions to which you should seek answers. Do you know the real reason the owner wants to sell? Has the salon been profitable? If not, do you know what will make it so? Are all the owner's records open and available to you? Is it debt-free and are there any outstanding liens on inventory or equipment and fixtures? Can any leases be transferred and are the terms of the lease favorable to you? Are there key people involved, such as busy stylists, and if so, what are their plans—to stay or leave? What guarantees are given? Will existing personnel sign noncompete agreements? As in any purchase of this sort, it is unwise to proceed without legal assistance. (Figure 1.2)

Buying an existing salon, even one you have worked in for a long time, more often than not may be an unsound idea. As our business is a largely personal one, when ownership changes hands, many times so does the clientele, even when the former owner leaves the area. There are many reasons for this, but know that this usually is the case. There is another consideration in buying an established salon, and that is your personal pride. No matter what you do, the business will probably always retain part of the former identity and not be wholly your own. If this would be nettlesome, reconsider.

The most important question you should ask when considering purchasing such a salon is could you open up next door with basically the same set-up and for basically the same price or lower? If you could, then there isn't much argument for buying such a business, is there? Often I think the reason stylists buy existing salons and pay far more than they're worth (they're worth chiefly the equipment value and

FIGURE 1.2
Purchasing an existing salon—should you or
shouldn't you?

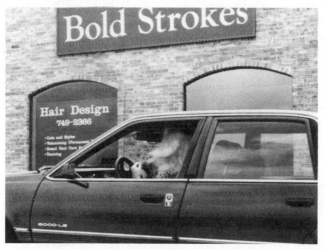

perhaps a favorable location value) is that they feel safer with an already proven commodity. If that is your reason for buying a salon, think twice. That is not a sound reason.

If you do decide to purchase an existing salon, by federal law you and the seller must file Form 8594 with the Internal Revenue Service. Usually, there are state and perhaps county or parish and/or city requirements as well. Contact your state attorney general and the secretary of state for more information.

OTHER PRE-OPENING ISSUES

Once you've decided how you're going to structure the business and if you're going to create a new salon or buy an already-existing one (or a franchise) you have made the first of what will seem (and are!) thousands of other decisions. And these must be made before you service the first client!

Contrary to what many may assume, business failures are not due to lack of business in most cases, but are caused by other easily controlled factors.

According to Larry Dietering, quoted in *Business Owner's Handbook*, published by Partners in Marketing, the nine most common causes of business failure are:

- Lack of experience
- Insufficient stock turnover
- Lack of business records
- Excessive accounts receivable
- Improper markup
- Inventory shrinkage
- Poor inventory control
- Inadequate financing
- Lack of sales

As you can see, eight of these can be managed through a structured accounting system. Therefore, the first rule of starting up a business is— get a good accountant! (That comes right after get a competent attorney.)

If you have never owned a salon before, don't despair. There are ways of learning to run a new business, even as you are setting it up or are in your first days of operation. Some of these ways, according to S. Nelton, in *Nation's Business* (reprinted in *Business Owner's Handbook*), are to:

- Hire smart people. You can learn from them, and they will help your business to grow and thrive. Many salon owners have admitted that their success was due to hiring smarter and more talented stylists than they. (Figure 1.3)
- Go to lunch! Eat out with those who know the things you don't about business—get into their heads and find out what they know.
- Continue your education, not only professional learning, but general business courses as well.
- Listen. Successful people listen to motivational or management tapes in the car.

FIGURE 1.3
Hire smart people!

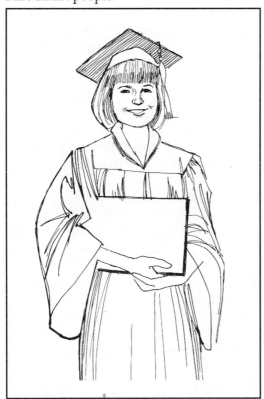

- Use the free services available. Educational meetings are sponsored by SBA, SCORE, ACE, SBDC, and others across the country (see Appendix A for lists of agencies).
- Trial and error. Making mistakes is part of the game—the trick is to learn from judgment errors so you don't repeat them.
- Join professional and business organizations. Chambers of commerce, trade associations, networking clubs, and other organizations provide significant learning experiences as you mix with other business owners. The acquaintances you make can also end up being clients.
- Work during lunch. Eat with your employees to stimulate better communication and creativity and solve problems.
- Listen to those close to you. Spouses, children, parents, and close friends all have valuable experience you can profit from. As they know your true strengths and weaknesses, and earnestly desire your success, discussing your business with them can be invaluable.
- Incubate or use executive office suites. Look at sites in the business enterprise zones that many cities provide for start-up and small businesses.
- Listen to your clients. Seek out from your customers what they perceive to be a weakness and what they see as a strength, so that you can either correct it or keep on doing the right things.

Other elements that can contribute to a successful start-up effort, according to an article by Gregory Monday in *Business Age*, are:

- Experience. Nothing beats what you already know. The two kinds of relevant experience are general business expertise and hairstyling experience. To be successful, both are necessary. If you do not have one of these (probably general business experience for most readers here, unless you are a layperson in the business strictly for the business opportunity), you will have to find it and pay someone to provide it to your salon. If, for instance, you have tons of styling experience but no business ability, one solution may be to bring aboard, as a partner, someone with the experience you lack.
- Responsibility. Take your responsibilities seriously. Know and understand your liabilities to clients, dependence on investors

and vendors, and exposure to state license boards and regulatory agencies. Proper acknowledgement and action toward responsibility brings you independence and control.

- Motivation and hard work. Get ready for the hardest job of your life! As a salon owner, you are now the organizer, owner, and manager as well as perhaps the bookkeeper, sales staff, advertising executive, receptionist, maintenance staff, and janitor! You will have to work long, hard hours and be paid only by the degree of success you are able to achieve in profitability. You must be motivated by the challenge and sense of achievement more than anything else.

- Optimism. Sadly, each year, thousands of salons fail. On the other hand, thousands make it. You may have such a failure yourself, before you become a success at owning a salon. It is not the end of the world—many successful owners have had major setbacks before they found the formula that worked for them. You must retain optimism for those inevitable periods of doubt.

- Objectivity. Egos loom large in our business, so make a concerted effort to keep yours under control. Having a distorted view of your talents, intuition, and importance can be fatal. Keep an open mind and realize that you don't know everything. When you come across information you don't agree with, don't ignore it—prove it wrong or gain a lesson from it.

- Mental and physical health. If you are in poor mental health, your motivation, optimism, and objectivity are affected. Keep things in perspective and strive for calmness in pressurized situations. Keep an eye on your mental "temperature." Your physical well-being is crucial for success as well. Long, hard hours of stressful work can take their toll. Be aware of possible health problems that can result, and take precautions or actions to alleviate the situation.

- Financial resources. You should not have to come up with all the funds for your venture yourself. Programs exist to aid the disadvantaged, and some private investors are interested in financing new businesses. Remember, however, each outside investor takes away part of your control, so the less outside assistance you require, the more control you retain.

THE FEASIBILITY STUDY

Just how feasible is your salon? That is one of the main questions you will need to answer before opening. Professional companies can perform feasibility studies for you, but they may be out of your price range. You can conduct your own feasibility study, and there are people who can help, such as the retired executives of SCORE, or perhaps your town or area has an active chapter of ACE (an organization of active business professionals who volunteer their expertise to start-up businesses).

The four errors made that disqualify feasibility studies and render them impotent are, "a lack of realistic goals and objectives, inadequate experience (including the ability to marshall all necessary resources at the level needed), failure to anticipate problems, and the inability to establish a market niche." (*Business Owner's Handbook,* Fall, 1990, available through the publishers, Partners in Marketing, 37 E. Ninth, Indianapolis, IN, 46204)

The feasibility study will lay the groundwork for the business plan (see chapter 2)—and should examine such areas, as taken from *Business Owner's Handbook,* Fall, 1990, as the business description, study of the competition, products and services to be offered, financial objectives, resources required, availability of a suitable location, executive and technical abilities, market study and sales projections, legal constraints, promotional plans, and much, much more.

According to *Starting Your Business* (Indiana Small Business Development Center, 1991), a feasibility study need not be unnecessarily complicated. It should clearly define the services and products to be offered; that the business will be founded on accurate assumptions; that the major contingencies have been provided for; that the owner has the proper experience and expertise to run the salon; and that the profit anticipated is enough to warrant the effort and resources the business will require.

There are excellent guides that offer more detail than in this overview. These are available through your local library, from the Small Business Administration, or from entities such as Small Business Development Centers and similar agencies and organizations to be found in most states.

THE BENEFITS OF CAREFUL PLANNING

The more research you can do and business knowledge you can accumulate prior to making a commitment to actually opening a salon, the better are your chances for survival and success. As you go through this text, make copious notes on everything that's unfamiliar to you, so that you can refer back when the information is needed. Refer to more elaborate sources when you need more comprehensive data than provided in this overview—many such sources are listed in the various chapters and especially in Appendix B. You will want to be like the football coach with the big game on Friday—you don't want to show up at the contest without the right equipment or a game plan—not if you expect to win the game! Planning properly ensures that your salon will still be around years from now and will be the one budding new owners will look to as a model of success and emulation.

Another important factor you will need to pay attention to is how you will manage your time. You will need to bring in income, of course, but you also must have sufficient time for training, bookkeeping, cash-flow management, promotion, supervision, and all the other duties required of the small business owner. Make a plan to have enough time to perform all the other jobs or you are asking for trouble. The days when all you had to do was work like a horse behind the chair and make money are over. Management skills are more necessary than ever, and to properly manage a salon, especially if you want to become bigger, will require that you sacrifice time spent behind the chair to devote to those duties. Even if you have no desire for your salon to grow very large, you still have to learn to maximize profitability, and to do so requires that you manage time properly and efficiently.

It is easy to become "married to the salon," and in a certain sense, this will happen, but it is important to realize that you should develop a life away from the business. Otherwise, your social and family life may suffer greatly, and you run the risk of becoming "burned out" and therefore a liability to the business itself! Many books and courses are available to help you if you have trouble effectively managing your time. Learn to set priorities and not be rigid with those priorities, but be able to re-prioritize as events transpire. Evaluate systems and methods that "buy you time," such as computer systems that help track clients, keep records, conduct inventory, do marketing surveys, and all the other time-consuming activities necessary to the efficient running of the salon.

Plan to delegate responsibility to others, especially lower-level activities at first, to free up your time for more important work. Just be sure you compensate for extra effort, and you will be building not only a stronger salon but a more motivated staff.

There is much to opening a hairstyling salon. Not only do you have to be an expert at the art and science of cosmetology, but you have to be well versed in business in general and small business in particular. You have not chosen an easy road perhaps, but it is a road that can lead to great financial rewards and enormous personal satisfaction. Your talent and the hard work you put forth will get you where you want to go, just as it has many others before you. Listen, learn, and heed the lessons of others who have shown the way to success, and when you have achieved your own goals, remember to look behind you and help those who are following the same road just traveled. If all of us give back to this great profession of beauty we practice, then we all will share in a stronger industry.

Let's get to work.

Good Luck!

REVIEW

Only proper planning will ensure that yours will be the one out of five new businesses that is still surviving five years from now. Three ways of structuring your salon are single proprietorship, partnership, and corporation. There are three types of salons: the specialty salon, the full-service salon, and the service and retail combination salon.

Whether you want to start a new salon or buy an existing one, you will need to answer a number of questions before you can decide if either is a good idea. The new business owner should ask for advice from both a competent attorney and a competent accountant. Information about starting a business can be obtained from a variety of places.

CHAPTER
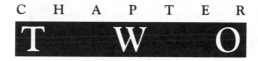

A business plan need not be complicated. Its sole purpose is to provide a guideline for what a business should be doing to become and remain profitable. It can be an instrument to steer the ship of business along often perilous waters, and it can be effective in obtaining start-up loans. Indeed, without such a plan to present, loaning agencies or individuals are less likely to seriously consider requests for funds. The properly designed plan is a powerful tool.

The failure rate of hairstyling salons is abysmally high. One of the chief reasons is that we, as stylists, approach business from a different perspective than many other small business owners. In many cases, we come into the entrepreneurial field from the artist's point of view, rather than from a solid business background. The common scenario is that a person graduates from cosmetology school, goes to work for a salon, and in three or four years achieves a full booking. At that time, the stylist begins to resent the commissions the owner is earning from his or her labor, and decides a better living can be obtained by opening his or her own salon *without any business expertise or knowledge.*

We sometimes are very naive about how businesses are operated. Too many times, new salon owners are fully booked with clientele, yet unable to generate a profit, or at least what should be a satisfactory profit. Business planning is the key that operates the door of success. (Figure 2.1)

FIGURE 2.1
Business planning is the key that opens the door of success.

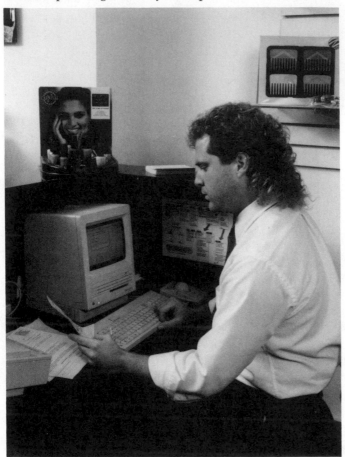

All businesses use some form of business planning, whether intended or not. After all, a business plan is simply a series of decisions that affect the business. It may be largely informal or very detailed and complex. The general rule of thumb is that the smaller the business the less formal and structured. A sound business plan should mirror the type of business it is designed for. Smaller businesses, such as most salons, tend to experience a more stable business environment; therefore, the plan may be relatively simple and provide for more flexibility. As the business becomes larger, the plan needs to become more comprehensive and complicated. For our purposes, it is assumed that the business plan will be for a small enterprise, of less than twenty employees. Larger businesses should seek a more comprehensive level of expertise than can be provided for here. Several publications are listed in Appendix B to help such businesses create an effective plan, and are recommended as well to smaller businesses that seek more thorough guidance.

Some of the uses of a good business plan are:

1. Identify strengths and weaknesses of the salon.
2. Improve performance of employees.
3. Give staff a clear picture of management's objectives and goals.
4. Measure the performance of the salon.
5. Provide a guide for decision making.
6. Provide for determining the effect of new developments on operations and strategies.
7. Educate and motivate staff.
8. Educate outside parties concerning the structure, performance, and objectives of a salon; this is essential when petitioning for a loan for either start-up purposes or expansion.

PARTS OF A SOUND BUSINESS PLAN

Experts generally agree that a sound business plan should contain five key elements. These are:

1. Marketing strategy
2. Organizational strategy
3. Financial strategy
4. Production and service strategy
5. Research and development or educational strategy

These five areas are what most business decisions should take into account, to some degree. Each is important, although, depending on the action being considered, some become more important. But each will probably be considered to some extent for any sound business decision.

Let's look at each area in general:

1. Marketing strategy—concerned with:
   A. Desirability of products and services to targeted segments.

    B. Preferences of clientele.
    C. Estimation of existing competition.

These three analyses help determine what can be sold to whom, when, how much, and at what price. A realistic estimate of these factors is crucial to the success of the salon. This area is of especial importance to potential investors, whether they be banks, credit unions, or other standard lending institutions, or private individuals or venture capitalists. Even a well-meaning and generous friend or relative prepared to invest in a salon will be grateful for such information before risking capital.

2. Organizational strategy
    A. Duties to be performed and who bears the responsibility for performing them.
    B. Organizing those duties for the best possible effectiveness, efficiency, and productivity.
    C. Staffing guidelines with a view to numbers of personnel, skill levels, and qualifications.
    D. Framework for guiding, motivating, and controlling overall operations of the salon.

Through this strategy, the salon manager decides how to put into practice the major business policies and plans. This will help determine who to put in charge and who will perform the various services needed to earn a profit and maintain the salon's smooth sailing.

Integrated into this part of the plan are evaluations of management's attitudes and philosophies for the salon, how employees are to be treated, and keystone markers of the salon's success. Also included are availability and cost of required staff to carry out the plan. Last, this section of the plan helps identify major strengths and weaknesses in the organizational structure, such as communication, cooperation, and morale and productiveness.

3. Financial strategy
    A. Cash flow
    B. Policies of the salon and supply houses regarding payments and collections.
    C. Performance of the salon on crucial financial indicators.
    D. Assets, liabilities, and future obligations.

E. Value and usefulness of assets.
F. Outside funds availability and cost.

This part of the plan is used to determine how the salon is to be managed to create a fair profit and ensure that the salon will remain in business. It also provides a plan for excess profits so they may be used wisely. The financial strategy is the litmus test for the other strategies of the business plan, satisfying such questions as: Does the current operation or planned operation provide a sufficient level of money to support the investment? Can the planned operation generate necessary cash flow to maintain the business atmosphere? Does the relationship of expenses and revenues maintain economic health?

4. Production and service strategy
   A. The process used to produce and deliver the salon's services and products.
   B. Facilities, materials, and equipment requirements.
   C. Schedule needed to support sales goals.

The purpose of a production strategy is simple. It determines the cost of producing the level of services and products necessary to achieve the established sales and revenue goals. The information gathered here is essential in determining the salon's breakeven point.

To determine these issues and develop a cohesive strategy, the following factors must be analyzed:

1. Production costs for each service and product.
2. Accurate estimation of lead time for obtaining products for resale.
3. Determination of supplier ability to provide products on time and with the required quality.
4. Determination of staff performance on services.
5. Evaluation of cost efficiency.

5. Research and development or educational strategy
As education is the cornerstone of competing effectively in today's salon business, a sound educational plan helps ensure success. Two areas need to be addressed when formulating this part of the plan. One, what are the crucial areas of the styling business the salon must maintain or expand for a competitive edge? Second, given future trends, what salon investment is needed to remain competitive?

Here is a good example of how the business plan can put your salon in the forefront, competitively. Let's say that you come from a salon that values education highly, and has made a practice of paying all the stylists' expenses to trade shows. You've seen the value of education by the quality of the work the returning stylists bring back with them. But you have a new salon and don't feel you can afford to send the three stylists you just hired to the big XYZ Show, and besides, there's the ABC Show coming up in just two more weeks. You have a brainstorm. Instead of sending all three stylists, as well as yourself, you pay the expenses of *one* stylist, with the proviso that the stylist conduct a class in the salon after returning from the show. And you decide to send another stylist to the ABC Show in two weeks, with the same plan. You realize you've covered two shows for two-thirds the initial cost, and now you find you can send yet a third stylist to the upcoming SOS Show in a month. You've covered three quality shows for the price of one.

This is all that a business plan does. Granted, you could have (and probably would have) come up with that idea without writing it down, as part of a formal plan, but the very act of putting a plan on paper seems to elicit such ideas more readily, and very definitely helps to fit them into the budget and overall scheme of the salon.

TIME PERIODS FOR PLANNING

For hairstyling salons, the most favorable time period to plan for is from one to two years. In some cases, you might wish to develop a five-year plan. Even if you feel you can conduct your business "in your head" and don't feel you need such a formal plan, there are some proven advantages to preparing such a plan, no matter how brilliant and business-wise you may be. It brings home the seriousness of planning; gives a framework to estimate future activities, past accomplishments, and possible opportunities; and forces the planner to provide objectives and strategies. The nature of our business has become so competitive that it is nearly impossible to survive without sound planning, no matter how talented a stylist one might be.

SAMPLE BUSINESS PLAN

The following is an example of how a business plan might look. Do not feel you have to imitate it, point by point, as your own needs might be more or even less complex. Rather, use it as a rudder by which to steer your own individual ship.

Publications are listed in Appendix B for those who are in need of a more comprehensive study of this subject. In particular, I can recommend the book put out by the American Management Association, *How to Write a Business Plan,* Second Edition, 1986. This volume may be found in your local library, or, if you should wish to purchase your own copy, the book is available by writing to the American Management Association, c/o Public Services, P.O. Box 319, Saranac Lake, NY, 12983, or by phoning (518) 891-5510. Current cost is $130 ($117 for members of that association). By the time this reaches print, they may have more current material available, so check. This may well be the wisest $130 ever spent for salon owners. It is comprehensive, detailed, and provides all the tools for putting together a business plan any lending institution or individual lender should ever require.

Below is an example of a general outline of what a properly designed business plan should include and look like. Depending on the business, in this instance the salon business, various sections can be de-emphasized or even deleted. Use your own judgment as to what a prospective investor may need or require, and decide what areas would be beneficial to you in providing a document that will help to steer your business and plan for the future wisely.

OUTLINE OF A BUSINESS PLAN DOCUMENT

I. Title page
  A. Name of firm
  B. Time period covered by plan
  C. Date of preparation
II. Table of contents
III. Executive summary
  A. The firm and its environment
  B. Current position and outlook
  C. Goals
    1. Financial
    2. Nonfinancial
  D. Strategies
    1. Marketing and sales
    2. Production
    3. Research and development
    4. Organization and management
    5. Finance
IV. Sales and revenue plan
  A. Sales and revenue objectives

  B. Product service line strategies
    1. Target customers
    2. Sales objectives
    3. Pricing policies
    4. Advertising, promotion
    5. Distribution
  C. Marketing and sales organization
V. Production plan
  A. Production schedule
  B. Production costs and standards
    1. Materials
    2. Labor
  C. Operating policies
    1. Inventory management
    2. Maintenance
    3. Purchasing
    4. Subcontracting
  D. Facilities
  E. Capital expenditures

continued

OUTLINE OF A BUSINESS PLAN DOCUMENT

VI. Research and development plan
    A. Assignment of responsibilities
    B. Management plan
        1. Objectives
        2. Expenses
VII. Organization and management plan
    A. Organizational structure
    B. Management policies and objectives
        1. General philosophy
        2. Recruitment and selection
        3. Training and development
        4. Compensation
    C. Position descriptions (if appropriate and needed)
    D. Resumes
VIII. Financial plan

    A. Schedules
        1. Income statements
        2. Balance sheets
        3. Cashflow summary
        4. Financial performance summary
        5. Departmental budgets
            a. Marketing and sales
            b. Production
            c. Research and development
            d. Administration
    B. Policies
        1. Debt management
        2. Investments
        3. Use of earnings
        4. Profit sharing

SOURCE: Reprinted from *How to Write a Business Plan,* Second Edition, American Management Association, 1986.

Title Page and Table of Contents

The document should have a title page that states the name of the firm, the time period covered or addressed by the plan, and final preparation date of the document. If the plan is to be used to raise funds, the time frame should be defined in terms of periods (year 1, first quarter, and so forth) rather than by specific dates. A table of contents follows the title page. The table of contents identifies each major section of the plan and the page number on which that section begins. If appropriate, a list of exhibits should also be included in the table of contents.

Executive Summary

In general, the executive summary presents an overview of the firm and the highlights of the completed business plan. Specifically, the executive summary should include the following subsections:

- The firm and its environment
- Current position and outlook
- Goals
- Strategies

The purpose of the executive summary is to present highlights and a brief but informative overview of what the firm is and where it is going. In general, the executive summary should not exceed five pages.

Sales and Revenue Plan

The sales and revenue plan identifies planned sales in terms of both units and revenue and outlines the basic marketing and sales strategy for achieving the planned sales levels. To be a useful management tool, the sales and revenue plan should describe the assumptions that underlie the marketing and sales objectives and decisions.

The description of the sales and revenue plan should include the following information:

- A schedule of quarterly or monthly and annual sales and revenue objectives differentiated, as appropriate, by product/service lines.
- A description of marketing strategy for each product/service line in terms of target customers, pricing strategy and discount policies, advertising and promotion efforts, and distribution networks.
- A budget for marketing and sales expenses differentiated, as appropriate, by product/service lines.
- An organization of marketing and sales responsibilities.

The description should also identify any plans for new product introduction during the period covered by the plan.

Production Plan

The production plan identifies production levels and outlines the basic strategy for achieving these levels. It should describe the assumptions that underlie the production objectives and decisions. The main assumptions are the cost of raw materials and production supplies, labor costs, and productivity standards. It should include the following information:

- A schedule of quarterly or monthly and annual production objectives differentiated, as appropriate, by product/service line.
- Productivity and production cost standards for each product/service line.

- Inventory policies for both raw materials and finished goods.
- Equipment utilization and maintenance policies.
- Production facilities.

The description should also identify any plans or requirements for capital expenditures related to plant and equipment.

Organization and Management Plan

The organization and management plan identifies the organizational structure of the salon and describes the salon's policies and standards for managing its human resources. It should include the following information:

- A statement of the salon's general management philosophy.
- An organizational chart.
- A description of authority and responsibility, or position descriptions for the various positions within the salon.
- Productivity measures and standards for the various positions within the salon.
- Policies and procedures for recruitment and selection of personnel, training and development, and compensation.
- Labor relations policies.

If the business plan has external uses (loan purposes), brief resumés of key personnel should also be included.

Research and Development Plan (Salon Personnel Education)

As appropriate and applicable, the research and development plan identifies the assignment of responsibilities for R&D activities and the budget for the period covered by the plan.

Financial Plan

The financial plan summarizes the expected financial performance and position of the salon as affected by the operations plans. The financial plan should include the following schedules that were developed through the planning process:

- Quarterly or monthly income statements.
- Quarterly or monthly balance sheets.

- Quarterly or monthly cash-flow summaries.
- Quarterly or monthly summaries of financial performance.
- Quarterly or monthly departmental budgets.

These financial schedules provide the framework for evaluating the financial viability of a salon's operations in both the planning and implementation phases.

The financial plan should also describe the policies of the salon for using financial leverage, evaluating investment opportunities, paying dividends (stock companies), and using excess cash.

Appendices

Most business plans should also include selected appendices that give more complete information that supports the plan. The specific nature and types of appendices vary, depending on the salon and the intended uses of the plan. For example, plans that are prepared in anticipation of raising funds should put detailed budgets in an appendix, rather than in the body of the financial plan.

The following is an example of a business plan for a fictional salon, designed not only as a planning document for establishing and running the business, but as an instrument in securing a loan. This is only intended to serve as a general guide; your own plan will need to be tailored for individual needs and may contain sections this plan omits, or may emphasize more heavily certain sections this plan does not. It is also intended to take the mystique out of such a plan. For those relatively uninitiated in business planning, this should serve as a friendly and nonthreatening outline for such an undertaking.

Business Plan
For a Company to Be Known As
Lagniappe Hair Design

Table of Contents—et al.
Executive Summary
 A. Our Company
      Lagniappe (Fr. something extra) Hair Design is to be a full-service salon, providing quality hair and skin services to an upscale and

---

Above descriptions excerpted from *How to Write a Business Plan,* 2nd ed.

discerning market. We will provide over twenty haircare quality product lines, as well as our own personalized line. Services to be offered include haircutting and styling, permanent waves (volumizers), all color and high-/low-lighting services, tanning, manicuring, sculptured nails and nail art, body wraps, therapeutic massage, a limousine service, depilation, and skin care and make-up.

There are to be two owners in a privately held enterprise, namely, Beau Smith and Delores Del Lores. Both are licensed cosmetologists and have a combined twenty years of experience in cosmetology and enjoy a full booking at Hair du Jour, where both are employed at present. Last year, Smith grossed service revenues for Hair du Jour in the amount of $81,000 and retailed $33,000 in product sales. Del Lores' figures were $76,000 and $38,000, respectively. Both expect to bring 100 percent of their patrons with them, as they are establishing their salon in the same general area, will be offering the same general prices, and the nature of their business is that they are both booked 100 percent by referral, not walk-ins.

The location chosen provides easy access, plentiful parking, is in an upscale neighborhood where the average household yearly income is $49,000, and is four blocks from their present place of employ. It is in a shopping center with a wide variety of services and goods, and enjoys a stable environment with less than 1 percent attrition rate among businesses over the past five years. It is widely recognized as the most vital shopping area in the city. The Cognetics Foundation lists the city as the fourth-best place in the United States for a start-up business of this kind to succeed. The Chamber of Commerce provides figures that estimate that up to 57 percent of the city's 250,000-plus population shop at this shopping center at least once annually, and the shopping center's own demographics record over a million and a half visitors to its stores and shops last year.

The current economy is in the midst of a prolonged upswing and citywide unemployment, while a remarkable 2 percent, is less than that in the local section, with out-of-work citizens accounting for less than 0.3 percent. Growth is predicted to be steady for the area, with much new construction and development ongoing. (See appendices for related charts.)

The customer base will be drawn from the following chief segments:

1. Women between the ages of eighteen and fifty-five.
2. Local neighborhoods, all ages.
3. Existing clientele.
4. Out-of-town and out-of-state clientele.
5. Professional and white-collar workers, predominantly women.
6. One-stop shoppers who would like to purchase a variety of haircare products at one place.

First-year goals are to establish service revenues of $173,000, which is a 10 percent increase above present combined earnings and a reasonable figure to aspire to. Retail sales goals are set at $78,000, which also allows for a 10 percent increase over the previous year's experience for both principals. It is fully anticipated that both incomes will be significantly higher, as additional personnel will be hired as expansion occurs. Retail sales should increase significantly more than provided for here, as it is planned to add six more product lines than were available at the former salon, and different marketing techniques will be employed as listed in the Sales and Revenue Section of this plan.

Strategies to achieve these goals include advertising on television and radio, allocating 5 percent of gross revenues to such advertising. The experience has been that to attract the clientele we have identified as favorable, television and radio represent the best buy for the dollar, giving the best return, and newspaper and other advertising provides a relatively poor return. We also plan to provide only a small yellow page ad and use that part of the advertising budget on more successful media. Yellow page ads look as though they would be worthwhile, but for our demographics, the cost exceeds the benefit. If we were a budget salon, such ads would probably be viable, but our demographic target can be better served with other forms of advertising.

We plan no "specials" or discounts on services. Such an act provides the wrong connotation to the image we are seeking to establish. From time to time, we plan to employ specials on retail items, chiefly in the form of "shrink-wrapping," and these will be planned around certain dates, such as holidays and other major buying periods.

Another strategy is to train personnel in effective prospecting and referral techniques.

Also, we will be aggressively selling tailored programs to fraternal organizations, social organizations, and business groups, where we will

deliver lectures and/or demonstrations on hair and fashion. The local cable
company has provided us with a time slot to air a weekly program on the
same subject, costing us nothing but our time. We also have contacted three
of the leading apparel salons to do the models' hair for their fashion shows,
as well as the leading bridal shop. We also provide a free blow-drying clinic
weekly, which our junior staff members will conduct, and from which we
anticipate booking a high percentage of new clients.

Sales and Revenue Plan

Objectives will be in terms of units sold, in the case of service
revenues. Retail items are sold at a mark-up of 50 percent. Our basic
units include (1) Haircut and styling, (2) Permanent wave, (3) Basic
coloring, (4) High-/low-lighting, and represent 85 percent of our service
revenues. Other services are not included in this summary, but are listed
in the Appendices, along with their unit price, selling price, and net
profit per service.

Unit cost for each service is determined as follows:

1. Haircut and styling—$5.45
2. Permanent wave—$11.90
3. Basic color—$7.35
4. High-/low-lighting—$9.10

These costs include basic raw materials and overhead. Percentages
or salaries paid to stylists are not added in at this time, and all costs are
predicted on an 80 percent booking schedule. While the two principal
owners are booked 100 percent, it is not to be expected that new
employees will be as busy.

Fees for each service are to be as follows:

1. Haircut and styling—$30
2. Permanent wave—$85
3. Basic color—$47
4. High-/low-lighting—$80

Haircuts account for approximately 50 percent of sales, permanents
25 percent, color 5 percent, and high-/low-lights 20 percent. Therefore,
to achieve our sales goals, the following minimum services must be sold
per month:

Haircut and Styling—231	=	$	6,930
Permanents—45	=		3,625
Color—15	=		705
High-/low-lights—37	=		2,960

Monthly total:	$ 15,220
	× 12 (mos.)
Yearly total:	$ 182,640

This does not include other stylists' income or revenue contributed, only the goals and projected revenues of the two owners. As stylists that are added will be recompensed on a percentage basis reflecting a figure that will provide a profit to the salon, those projections are not included for these purposes.

Production Plan

Production costs for salon services are firmly fixed and predictable, allowing, of course, for normal price increases from suppliers. Such increases will be reflected immediately in charges made for services to the client, thereby not placing the business at a disadvantage.

Whenever possible, and whenever an attractive price is available, stock purchases will be made, taking into account cost of storage, cost of monies so invested, etc. Educational events usually present such opportunities, as dealers traditionally offer deals, which will be fully taken advantage of. Also, bulk rates will be sought among all suppliers, again using the aforestated formula in determining if the buy would be advantageous.

Equipment will be maintained in excellent condition, for attractiveness, ease in working, and the salon image. Insurances will be provided on all major equipment. It is planned to remodel extensively every three years, replacing some major equipment and refurbishing others, i.e., re-covering styling chairs. Walls and floors will be remodeled every four years, creating a new decor.

Inventories will be taken on a weekly basis, accounting for all use supplies as well as retail supplies.

Each product line will be tracked as to profitability. Unprofitable lines will be replaced by those deemed more profitable only after all efforts are made to increase sales by aggressive marketing, rearrangement of placement, etc.

Organization and Management Plan

All management policies and procedures are as outlined in the salon employees' handbook, which is included in the Appendices. In general, we promise to provide a safe, attractive environment in which to practice the trade of cosmetology, and provide a fair wage in return for an honest day's labor. We expect all employees to maintain a standard of excellence based and set forth upon their position, and to assist in all phases of a smooth salon performance. Cleanliness and neatness are paramount, not only in the salon itself, but in personal hygiene and dress. Dress codes are strictly enforced. Employees must dress fashionably at all times, and that definition is at the discretion of the owners. Further details can be found in the handbook.

Organizational chart:

1. Owners—Smith and Del Lores
2. Salon Coordinator
3. Designers and Specialists
4. Co-Designers

Position Descriptions:

1. Owners

The owners provide the basic policies, goals, and direction for the salon. All rules, standards, prices, and codes are determined by the owners. Salon goals and the procedures to achieve those goals are set forth by the owners. Final decisions on all aspects are their domain; however, authority in certain areas is designated to those subordinate, as provided. The owners are responsible for maintaining the integrity and image of the salon, as well as its profitability.

2. Salon Coordinator

The "quarterback" of the salon, this person is responsible for managing the day-to-day running of the business and carrying out and implementing the owners' decisions and policies. In addition, the salon coordinator acts as the chief receptionist and assists in the bookkeeping functions as designated. The salon coordinator shouldn't be involved in the technical aspects of cosmetology, although the person may have cosmetology training. She is the manager and does the weekly purchasing and disbursements, at the direction of the owners. Disputes within the salon should be brought to the salon coordinator, and to the owners only as a last resort. Remunerated at an agreed-upon salary and various benefits the salon can provide, he or she is also on a bonus system that is tied to overall profitability. The salon coordinator arranges employees' schedules and disburses payroll checks.

3. Designers and Specialists

These are the senior technical members of the staff, and provide leadership and skills for the rest of the salon. Their prices are the highest, reflecting the quality of their work and skill. They provide training to co-designers and a desirable role model. Specialists are on the same level and are those persons who specialize in make-up, skin care, body wraps, and other specialized salon services. These positions are not taken lightly, nor are they given lightly. To earn the designation of designer or specialist, an employee must follow a prescribed formula to attain the position, as outlined in the employee handbook. No one is hired initially as a designer, no matter what the person's talent or client base. Everyone in the salon must appreciate the work and diligence co-designers must adhere to, so that they can treat those persons with respect and dignity. Designers and specialists are allowed to raise their prices commensurate with their booking schedule, again according to the formula found in the handbook. In effect, the only ceiling on their fees is the fullness of their personal booking. They also serve as the instructors in the weekly educational classes held for co-designers and other personnel. (Figure 2.2)

4. Co-Designers

Co-designers are ordinarily the newer employees. They are to assist designers and all other personnel in the salon. They maintain the cleanliness of the salon, meet and greet clients as soon as they enter the premises, offer clients refreshments, maintain the tanning bed and the scheduled appointments, make the coffee, run errands, do the laundry, and assist in whatever ways other salon personnel request. They also provide co-designer client services at co-designer prices, which are lower, and further their education at every opportunity by viewing videotapes, attending the weekly educational meetings, attending shows and events, and simply observing designers as they work. They are required to achieve certain levels at certain time frames, and if they do not achieve those levels, they may be dismissed. It is an apprenticeship position, designed to be a learning experience for them.

The philosophy behind our "level" system of designers is twofold. First, it protects the client from paying too much for service given by one who is not yet qualified to provide work up to the salon standard. Second, it protects the new stylist from having to try to perform at a level

FIGURE 2.2
Designers at all levels continue to learn.

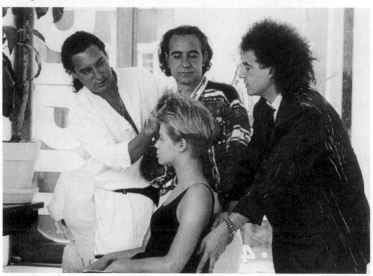

he or she is simply not ready to perform at. It also provides a quality service at a more affordable price for those unable to pay premium prices, as we believe our co-designers are the equivalent of the average designer in other salons in our city. Even our lowest level designers are not permitted to service clients until they have satisfactorily passed our basic salon training program. At that time, they are carefully monitored as to what services they can perform and on whom. We feel it is simply the most equitable system designed for those on either side of the styling chair.

Research and Development Plan (Salon Education)

We are firmly dedicated to the principle of educating ourselves and our employees. We already have an extensive library of videotapes that will be required viewing for all employees, upon which they are to be tested. We also hold an in-salon educational meeting once weekly, in which our designers provide instruction for our co-designers. To further make use of available educational funds in our budget, we will send, at salon cost, one employee to each show, with direction that that person is to return and pass on to us what he or she has learned. In that way, we will be able to attend a great many more shows and events than if we were to send everyone, as is commonly done.

Financial Plan

The financial plan will include the following monthly reports: income statements, balance sheets, cash-flow summaries, financial performance summaries, and budgets.

These reports, prepared in conjunction with our accountant, will also be furnished to any lending institution or individual who has invested in us, and will be the basis of determining if we are on track to achieve our stated goals, and if not, how to pinpoint weaknesses we might not be aware of so that we might correct them.

Appendices

This should include any and all of the documents mentioned in the body of the overall plan. This one does not, as it is a purely fictional plan, but plenty of examples of what should be included are given.

If the plan is also to be used as a tool in obtaining loans, a separate section should be attached, explaining in detail the monies sought and for what purpose they will be used. Your accountant should be able to help you list those things in which a lending institution or individual would be interested. In general, they should include the amount of the loan, the location, cost of leasing or buying, equipment cost, stock cost, suppliers and vendors to be used; in other words, every single item the money is to be spent on and what it will cost. You should also list the cost of operation, including debt service, and show what your breakeven point will be and what it will take to achieve that point.

Don't make the mistake of underestimating costs involved in establishing and operating a business and overestimating anticipated revenues. Any reasonable financial person will spot such attempts readily, and besides, you do yourself no service when you figure on pie-in-the-sky as expected good fortune. Allow yourself plenty of latitude in determining the funds necessary to proceed; investors will see you as a prudent business person. By the same token, don't try to provide for every contingency imaginable. There does exist an element of risk in any business—that's why lenders make the big bucks! Figure high on expenses and reasonably low on revenues, and make the potential lender aware that's what you've done. If you honestly have reason to believe you have grossly underestimated the business' capacity, inform the lender of that without overstating the case. As in all dealings, just be as honest as you can and state your case plainly.

Seek out professionals for their assistance. Your accountant should be a working partner in all planning, and very possibly legal aid would also be desirable. Don't try to skimp on expenses by doing your own tax work or any serious financial planning. A good accountant will save you far more than he or she will ever charge, even though that fee may seem high at the time.

Even if you aren't in need of a loan for your business, whether for start-up or expansion, if you don't already have a business plan in effect, take the steps to create one. It will show you, at the very least, how to make the salon more productive and profitable—and that's the bottom line!

REVIEW

The purpose of a business plan is to act as a guideline for what a business should do to become and remain profitable. The most favorable time period for planning is one to two years, although sometimes an owner might wish to develop a five-year plan.

A sound business plan contains five key elements: a marketing strategy, an organizational strategy, a financial strategy, a production and service strategy, and an educational strategy.

C H A P T E R

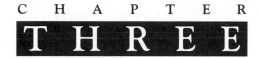

The first thing that should be determined before opening a salon is whether you have the necessary skills and experience that will be required of a salon owner. This may seem unnecessary, but some people who want to open a business are grossly underqualified to do so and make a success of it.

The first step is to take an inventory of yourself and your motives for opening a salon in the first place. If your overriding reason for wanting your own place is that you hate your boss and where you currently work, you may want to reevaluate your decision and see if you'd be better off searching for a new job instead. Owning a business is a serious commitment that will require a lot of long, hard hours, and you may not succeed in spite of everything. This is not to discourage anyone from opening a salon, just those who may be doing so for the wrong reasons. Being prepared in all ways, which includes mentally, is crucial to any chance of success, and with some individuals, it may be wiser to delay opening a salon until a later date.

Take stock of yourself. Ask these questions.

1. What is my motivation for opening a salon?
2. What level of training and skill do I possess compared to other salon owners with whom I will be competing?

3. What are the most difficult problems I face now as a stylist employed in a salon? Do I think those problems will diminish as an owner? Why?

4. What economic and personal prices am I prepared to pay?

5. What are my strengths and weaknesses? What do I do well, and what do I like doing?

6. How much money can I invest, whether my own or borrowed? Will it be possible to attract or borrow the additional funds needed to open my business?

7. Would I be satisfied with less control if any investors require this?

8. How much do I need to make this year? Next year? The next five years? Ten years?

9. What considerations other than financial motivate me?

10. What support do I have from family and friends?

11. Will I run the business or hire a manager? Am I able to delegate authority?

12. How much time can I invest in the business on a week-to-week basis and be happy?

13. How well can I handle stress?

14. Do I enjoy what I do as a stylist? (This is perhaps the most important thing to ask yourself. If you don't like styling hair, but you think the income you anticipate making as an owner will offset your dislike, then you are making a grave mistake and would probably be better off thinking about a career change.)

These are just a few of the questions to honestly answer about yourself before you begin looking at the ways and means of opening your salon. If you can look inside and answer most of these questions positively, then it's time to roll up your sleeves and get to work! Various chapters in this book offer clear methods to achieve such things as obtaining loans, purchasing equipment, performing inventory, hiring and training personnel, and all the other thousand and one components a viable business requires. To help you determine when, where, and how to open your salon, enlist the aid and assistance of everyone you can. You know the craft of hair—now it's time to learn the craft of operating a small business. Addresses and phone numbers for many of the organizations listed below may be found in Appendix A.

INFORMATION SOURCES

The Small Business Administration (SBA) is a very helpful resource with a variety of services, including information, financial assistance, and hands-on help through the offices of the Service Corps of Retired Executives (SCORE). Funded by the SBA, SCORE is designed to help small business owners such as yourself with expert advice and information from experienced business persons. They maintain offices in each state of the United States, and may be found in the phone book under Federal Government.

Colleges and universities can be very helpful, offering many courses of interest and use to the small business owner.

Competitors are one of the best sources of information available. Very few trade secrets are left anymore. Seek out people outside of your geographic area for advice, and you will be surprised at the information they are usually willing to impart. Even many of those within your area have no problem with advice.

Most states maintain economic development offices either at the capital or located in major cities in your state, offering valuable information and assistance to start-up businesses such as yours.

Chambers of commerce are excellent sources, located in most cities of any size. They work with government, education, financial, and business groups and can bring that expertise to assist you. This is usually a very good organization to join, not only for the aid and succor available to you as a business owner, but for the social and networking activities and the lobbying clout that can be helpful to small businesses. Most chambers also maintain very good libraries of business references, available to members.

Don't forget libraries themselves as a free, convenient resource with information about demographics, industry trends, projected growth of areas, and general business.

Trade associations are extra valuable resources when planning a salon, because of their specialized knowledge. Organizations such as the National Cosmetology Association (NCA) are excellent. Local hairdressers' guilds, both of national affiliation or state, may offer the best information you can find anywhere.

Gain all the information about business in general and small and salon business in particular.

One word of caution. If you are anticipating purchasing an already-existing salon, you by all means should have an attorney, and make use of The Uniform Commercial Code Bulk Transfer Act, which applies to practically all businesses. When a seller transfers a major portion of the business inventory, supplies, and equipment, a bulk transfer takes place. Following the aforenamed law will protect you from commercial fraud schemes, such as the seller leaving you with unpaid debts.

MARKET RESEARCH

However you plan to establish your business—either by purchasing an existing salon or by creating a new one—the first thing you should do is market research. You have to find out if there are any clients out there—at least enough to make opening your business worthwhile.

These are the questions you should try to answer:

1. Are your styling services and retail items wanted?
2. How many potential clients are there?
3. What will they pay for your services and products?
4. Is this number on the rise or declining?
5. Where do your potential clients live?
6. What are their ages and incomes?
7. What else do you know about them?
8. What are their buying motivators?
9. What do they value?
10. How would your location affect this clientele?
11. From what geographical population would you draw?
12. What are its size and traffic patterns?
13. Is this projected clientele enough to support your business?
14. How many competitors will there be?

Demographics are useful in predicting success. You need to know not only who your customers are or will be, but where they live and work and how much they will spend for your services.

A host of factors weigh into the market share. Income levels, age groups, sexes, buying habits, should all be quantified and studied. You will need to know neighborhood make-ups, traffic patterns, growth patterns of both residential and commercial areas in your proximity, economic forecasts for both the segment you wish to serve and also the area in which you will operate. You will also want to determine the strength of support and supply groups, such as banks, transportation systems and arteries, suppliers, availability of staff personnel, and so on.

Product dealers are excellent sources of such information. They have the expertise to advise what areas will support what kinds of salons and can point out mistakes you may commit before they are made. If, however, your plan is to open a type of salon not normally seen in your area, but which you have good reason to believe will succeed, be sure to weigh carefully any adverse advice against your other data.

If, for the sake of argument, you decide to open an upscale salon in a town that so far has not had such an enterprise, but you see a good chance for success based on the numbers of people who go out of town for that level of service, some advisors may frown on your plan. Listen to them, for they may be aware of factors you aren't, but there is also the chance that they are in error in their judgment. In such a case, gather as much information as you can to support your premise and base your strategy on that. The American system of free enterprise allows for such gambles, and when they pay off, they pay off handsomely. The more information you can glean, the more businesslike decisions you will be able to make and the better your chance for survival and/or prosperity. Keep in mind that pipe dreams rarely come true outside of the movies. Back up projected goals with solid research and not wishful thinking.

Your research, for example, may reveal that 10 percent of the population of your town of 50,000 travels sixty miles on a regular basis to the sort of salon you envision. That kind of knowledge may tell you that although there hasn't been a salon of this type in the area before, an identifiable and sizeable portion of the market desires such a salon and travels a long distance to obtain those kinds of services. These are the types of data you should be looking for. It is not enough to simply accumulate a mass of facts and figures; once you have them, you must make some sort of sense out of them and apply what you learn to your planning.

Information about competitors is also important. Look through the phone book and note their locations. Even drop in on them and see how they conduct business. You don't have to announce what you are doing or who you are. Get your hair styled or buy a bottle of shampoo—and observe! Note the types of clients they seem to be serving.

Research to determine the maximum amount your clients will pay for your services and products. Determine if a higher price will increase profits or decrease sales, and if a decrease in prices would increase sales volume enough to increase your profit. Market research is necessary to determine these decisions.

You will also need to research what is the best marketing plan. What kind of advertisements are most cost effective in terms of return on investment? You should also know how your competitors' marketing efforts are working. You can do your own research or even hire companies that conduct primary and secondary marketing research. Begin immediately to collect rate cards and demographic information from those trying to sell advertising to you. You can use these rate cards and other information to rough out a marketing budget and timetable for your own advertising and marketing.

Like it or not, this is the age of automation and the computer. Once a pricey toy and a luxury, computers and salon software systems are fast becoming a necessity for the salon that desires to stay up with the competition. More about computers can be found in other chapters in this book, and it is highly advisable to gain as much knowledge and education in this area as possible. Prices for both computers and software systems are becoming extremely reasonable, as is ease of operation. If you are completely computer illiterate (as all of us were at one time) there are a lot of inexpensive ways to gain an education. Start writing to the manufacturers of the systems that advertise in the salon trade journals and magazines. The right software can save you time and money in any area of the salon business.

LOCATION

Once you have done your market research and compiled your business plan, you are ready to begin looking for a location.

Someone once asked a successful business person what he considered the three most important factors for success in business, and he replied, "That's easy! Location, location, location!" This is a twist on the old advertising person's answer to the same question, but there is a very large kernel of truth to it. (Figure 3.1)

FIGURE 3.1
The three most important factors in opening a new salon are:
Location, Location, and Location!

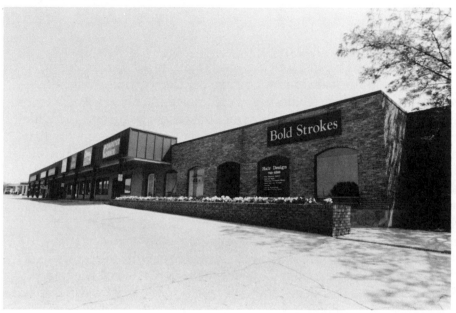

Without the best possible location, the new salon owner faces an uphill battle, and, while some salons may prosper without a great deal of advertising, excluding word-of-mouth referrals, salons enjoying a vigorous rate of traffic located in poor locations are almost nonexistent. To be sure, there are exceptions, but if such a weed happens to grow in rocky soil, it may be safely assumed that it would grow even bigger and faster in a better climate and surroundings.

The location of your salon can literally determine its success or failure. Consider factors such as possible inconvenience that might occur to clients from being on one-way streets, or if they will be forced to make left-hand turns into your parking lot, or the amount and kinds of insurances the owner may require—all these and other factors may have a significant impact on your business. Other considerations when selecting a location are the level and kind of services to be offered, the initial size of the business—both physical size and quantity of personnel—and the demographics of the target market. The amount of capital required and/or available will contribute to the decision as well.

Helpful aids are Small Business Administration publications *Management Aids #2.002—Locating or Relocating Your Business,* or *MP10— Choosing a Retail Location.* (See Appendix A for addresses.)

Assessing the Competition

Selecting a location should begin with assessing the competition you are comfortable vying against for your market share. This can be done in various ways. One method is to obtain a detailed city map of the area you are contemplating (chambers of commerce usually have such maps available). Identify existing salons from the yellow pages and mark them on the map. You can use colored pins and rank them according to their type. For instance, if you classify the salon you are opening as an upscale salon, you might want to identify all such salons with a blue pin. You could choose a red pin for salons you'd consider budget salons, and a white pin for those that fall in between. You may wish to identify other classifications or categories of salons and use different color pins to exhibit barber shops or men-only styling salons.

Laying this out on a map gives a real idea of what the competition looks like, and it is easy from such an exhibit to visualize the layout. Sometimes, areas previously unthought of as potential sites will leap out at you when this is done.

If you do not anticipate the majority of your business coming from a neighborhood clientele, this may not warrant the time. However, if you expect and want to draw clients from the area in which you operate, this will be a valuable exercise.

Assuming you do want to draw from the surrounding area, the next step is assessing your competition. Perhaps you have practiced your trade long enough in the area to have a good handle on the salons you will be competing against, but even so, it may be a wise move to investigate more thoroughly. JeriSue Petry and Time Temporary Services, a services industry specializing in filling employment needs, provided the Competitor Assessment Guide (Figure 3.2) to assist in evaluating your competition. It has been amended to better suit the salon business and, if utilized properly, may be of enormous aid in seeing how your proposed salon stacks up against competing salons.

Much of the information in the Competitor Assessment Guide you may obtain yourself, by simply visiting salons and asking for information. Some you can garner from your own knowledge of each

FAR-AHEAD STYLING SALON   **COMPETITOR ASSESSMENT GUIDE**

Prepared by _____ Date _____

COMPANY INFORMATION

Company_____ Owner/Manager_____

Address _____

Contact_____ Title _____ Phone #_____

Staff members _____ Receptionists _____ Stylists _____ Colorists _____

Perm technicians _____ Make-up artists and Skin-care specialists _____

Levels of designers _____ Support personnel _____ Retail specialists _____

Other (specify)_____

Length of time in business_____ At this location_____

Type of operation: _____ Franchise   _____ Individual   _____ Partners

_____ Corporation _____ Other (Specify)

Services offered: _____ Haircutting _____ Color   _____ Perming

_____ Make-up & Skin care _____ Massage

_____ Body wraps _____ Nail care   _____ Other

GENERAL INFORMATION

What are the advantages of using your salon services? _____

_____

What are your office hours? _____

What makes your salon different from others?_____

Services offered	Skill level	Rate	% Paid to empl.
_____	_____	_____	
_____	_____	_____	
_____	_____	_____	
_____	_____	_____	
_____	_____	_____	

FIGURE 3.2
Competitor assessment guide (*continued on next page*).

FAR-AHEAD STYLING SALON   **COMPETITOR ASSESSMENT GUIDE**

Employee Benefits

Benefit	Yes	No	Explanation
Holiday pay	_____	_____	_____
Vacation pay	_____	_____	_____
Sick pay	_____	_____	_____
Hospitalization	_____	_____	_____
Life insurance	_____	_____	_____
Referral bonus	_____	_____	_____
Pay raises	_____	_____	_____
Other _____	_____	_____	_____
_____			

Physical Facility

Description of area (business, commercial, residential) _____

Access to public transportation _____

Description of: Outside of building _____

Entrance/Lobby _____

Description of salon (layout, size, # of rooms, decor) _____

_____

_____

Equipment in salon _____

_____

Comments _____

_____

_____

FIGURE 3.2
Competitor assessment guide.

salon's reputation. Another way of obtaining information is to have someone unknown to the salon visit it, perhaps on the pretext of obtaining employment or as a potential client. Should you think this is somehow immoral, you will, of course, have to let your own conscience be your guide, but you should be aware that many businesses of all kinds routinely perform such investigations prior to investing large sums of capital on their own locations. Most consider it merely a prudent business measure.

If you feel you can obtain the information needed by simply asking and being honest about your motives, be sure to thank the manager or owner for his or her time and send a thank-you note promptly. If you choose a person to collect the information, you should be certain he or she understands the information you want to obtain. When conducting the assessment, the individual should observe very closely and gather as much information and promotional material as possible, filling out a report as soon as possible after the visit or phone call. The type of information gathered will include the quality of salon personnel, the types and quantities of services offered, pricing structure, methods of obtaining and retaining clientele, educational programs within the salon, pay scales (including benefits to employees), and how personnel are obtained and retained.

Determining Space Requirements

When determining space requirements, consult several of your local product dealers for recommendations, providing them with details they will need, such as services to be offered, number of employees, and plans and timetables for expansion. Office design companies may be valuable for recommendations as well, but normally most dealers are more familiar with space requirements for our industry.

When selecting possible sites, it is important to understand how the cost of office space is determined. Office space pricing is determined, first of all, by its location. Downtown business districts, depending on the town, may be more expensive than comparable space in suburban areas, due to parking and public transportation access. Shopping malls may be more expensive yet. The condition and age of the building are also factors. Various standard ways of leasing space are listed here from the most expensive to the least:

- Turnkey office space in which the lessor prepares the space to fit your needs and absorbs the costs of taxes, maintenance, and janitorial services.
- Improved space in which you and the lessor negotiate modifications and maintenance costs.
- Raw space in which you bear the cost of all modifications and maintenance.

Office space terms are usually quoted as annual rent per square foot. For example, a space of eight hundred square feet that rents for $10 per square foot would cost $8,000 per year. To compute the monthly rate, simply divide $8,000 by twelve to arrive at $667.

The square footage of space is usually calculated as the distance from the middle of one interior wall to the middle of the opposite interior wall, multiplied by the distance from the inside of the wall dividing the office from the hallway to the inside of the wall dividing the office from the outside.

SITE ASSESSMENT

Prior to visiting sites, you should have a clear price range in mind. When you visit, take a tape measure to measure the dimensions yourself. Although most would not intentionally mislead you, space may not be measured uniformly by the owner and/or realtor.

To select a good location, you should use various criteria and resources, as well as your own personal knowledge of the area. Chamber of commerce personnel can help you identify price ranges and advantages of the various high-traffic areas in the business and suburban districts. A salon in the business district has the advantage of being convenient to other businesses and can encourage walk-in clientele. A salon in a suburban area may attract customers from both the surrounding business and residential areas.

Call several realtors and let them know what you are looking for. Target areas that provide high traffic, but where there is little competition. You should be able to locate these areas by using the map you marked for your Competitor Assessment Guide.

The Site Assessment Guide (Figure 3.3), adapted from a similar one Time Temporary Services uses, will help you gather the information you need to better select a good location and negotiate your lease. Visit potential locations and record your observations on this form, for a guide in determining the best possible location.

When assessing locations, heed the following factors:

External factors. As you approach the building, note:

- Visibility of the address on the building.
- Access to public transportation. (This may be unimportant, depending on your targeted clientele.)

FAR-AHEAD STYLING SALON   **SITE ASSESSMENT GUIDE**

Developer _____ Phone # _____

Address _____ Floor/# Location _____

Total square feet _____ Cost per aquare foot_____

Landmarks _____

Traffic patterns _____

Services in building or provided _____

Nearest salon of comparable quality _____

EXTERNAL FACTORS	OK As Is	Needs Some Work	Needs Major Work	Questions/ Comments
Address visibility				
Ease of entrance				
Access to public transportation				
Parking space/ lighting				
Condition of parking lot				
Condition of sidewalks				
Landscaping				
BUILDING CONDITIONS				
Facade/Entrance				
Lobby				
Elevator/Stairs				
Hallways				
Floors				
Walls/Partitions				
Windows/Glass				
Blinds/Drapes				
Lighting/Fixtures				
Rest rooms				

FIGURE 3.3
Site assessment guide *(continued on next page).*

FAR-AHEAD STYLING SALON   **SITE ASSESSMENT GUIDE**

	OK As Is	Needs Some Work	Needs Major Work	Questions/ Comments
OFFICE REQUIREMENTS				
Sign Visibility/ Condition				
Office Layout				
Air Cond./Controls				
Heat/Controls				
Soundproofing				
Elec. Outlets				
Lighting Fixtures				
Telephone Jacks				
Storage				

Utilities/ Maintenance	Cost Per Month	Install Cost	How Service Is Measured
Air conditioning			
Electric			
Heat			
Janitorial service			
Maintenance			
Telephone			
Trash removal			
Water			

Maintenance Service	How Often	Paid for By

Janitorial Service	How Often	Paid for By

FIGURE 3.3
Site assessment guide (continued on next page).

FAR-AHEAD STYLING SALON	SITE ASSESSMENT GUIDE
How often is the facility painted	*Not included in Maintenance/ Janitorial Services*
on the inside? _____	_____
on the outside? _____	_____
Are touch-ups done	_____
per request? _____	_____
YES _____ NO _____	_____

FIGURE 3.3
Site assessment guide.

- Lighting features and condition of the parking lot.
- Condition of the sidewalks.
- Landscaping and maintenance of the grounds.

Ask yourself, "Does this place look well maintained, and is it an easy and convenient place to get in and out of? Does it look like the kind of exterior decor my clients will appreciate and find attractive?"

Parking. A major consideration should be proximity to easily accessible parking for clients. Parking should also be adequate for your staff as well. Figure two and a half times your maximum client load at the busiest time, to allow for stylists running behind, early-arriving clients, or walk-ins for services or retail items. If an area does not provide adequate parking space, seriously consider looking elsewhere.

Building facade and entrance. When a prospective client or employee visits your salon, the first impression he or she will have of your business will be determined by the facade of the building. Ask yourself if the facade and entrance to the building represent the quality with which you want to be associated.

Office location within the building. It is preferable to have an office on the first floor of a building due to its visibility and accessibility. If this is not possible, the next preference is to select a space within direct eyesight of the elevator or stairwell. An obvious exception to this is if your city has a status address in a high-rise, but to build a volume business, even these sites are usually not desirable.

Lobby and hallway. The second impression a prospective client or employee will have of your salon, should you choose to locate in a business building, will be formed from the condition and decor of the lobby and hallways. Are they in good condition, clean, well lighted, and pleasantly decorated?

Stairs and elevators. Stairs and elevators should be in good condition, well lighted, and above all, safe.

Soundproofing. If your space is close to other businesses, it will require soundproofing to ensure the comfort of your clients. Adequate soundproofing is possible with insulated snap-in walls, or an insulated wall placed between two outer drywall panels. Be careful of walls that are insulated only up to the ceiling. You can determine how far a wall is insulated by pushing up the ceiling tile and looking into the area next to a dividing wall. Because of the sometimes unpleasant odors associated with our business, i.e., permanent waves and nail preparations, be sure that those odors will not cause a problem for other adjacent businesses. I once had a salon in a racquetball club and had already signed a lease and purchased equipment when the manager of the club decided the salon should not be in the closed space we had agreed to, but in an open space. As I was already committed, I felt I had no choice but to acquiesce. We enjoyed a good business, but it would have been so much more enjoyable, and probably better for business, if we didn't constantly overhear stage whispers about "What's that horrible smell?"

Heating and air conditioning. Controls for each should be in your space rather than in another area of the building. If this is not the case, but the space meets your other requirements, ask that the present policies regarding control of heating and air conditioning be mentioned in your lease. If there are no policies, request to have an agreement regarding heating and air conditioning control written into your lease.

Telephone capabilities. You will need sufficient telephone jacks, conveniently placed for your reception area and other areas where phones are needed, as well as the capacity to add other lines later. If you are going to use a computer, be sure the existing telephone lines can be used as computer data lines.

Electrical outlets. Be sure there are plenty of outlets for all your dryers, clippers, and other electrical apparatus, including washers and dryers. If you plan to use equipment requiring a different voltage, such as 120 amps for tanning beds, be sure such is available. Be certain plenty of outlets will be available should you decide to remodel in the future.

Leasehold improvements. Determine what improvements or modifications need to be made to create the environment you desire. Analyze the layout and space to see if there will be sufficient work space, retail space, office space, or whatever additional needs you may have. If there is insufficient storage space, for instance, you may want to add these improvements to your lease.

Janitorial and maintenance services. Check the rest rooms! They are one of the best signs of quality maintenance and janitorial service. They will tell you the care the rest of the building or mall receives. Check the condition of the floors, walls, carpets, and windows. Find out who is responsible for maintenance and janitorial services and if any of those services are provided.

NEGOTIATING A LEASE

You've done your homework and arrived at the best possible location, but you're not done yet. You don't want to just sit down and sign whatever lease the landlord puts in front of you, at least not normally. It is time to do some negotiating; clarify the terms of the lease. A Lease Checklist (Figure 3.4) is provided to assist you and provide guidance during the negotiating period. Some of the things you will want to talk about and get settled in writing are:

Option to sublet. Insist that your lease state your right to sublet the space should you need more room. If no more space is available in the same building, you should have the right to move where you can grow.

Noncompete clause. Require that your lease include a section preventing another similar salon from renting in your building or area owned by the same company, such as in a mall, unless you deem the mall is large enough to support other salons of the same quality as yours. If the lessor balks at such a clause, ask to put in a clause that would nullify your obligation to the lease should another salon of similar quality lease space in your proximity.

Heating and air conditioning. If the controls are not in your space, make an agreement describing the temperature control and add it to the lease. Also, clarify how the electricity will be measured and who pays for it.

Signs. Clarify the type of sign allowed and lettering and copy allowed. We had a situation arise once in which we had signed the lease

FAR-AHEAD STYLING SALON   **LEASE CHECKLIST**

COSTS

Monthly rent	$ _____
# Square feet	_____
Cost per sq. ft.	_____
Security deposit	_____
Monthly taxes	_____
Other deposits	_____
Other expenses	_____
Total	$ _____

TERMS

Date lease to begin	_____
Length of lease	_____
Option to renew at same rate	_____
Option to sublet	_____
First choice on additional space	_____
Noncompete clause	_____
90-day cancellation notice	_____
Contingency clause	_____

All lease terms are in writing and have been reviewed by my lawyer.

Signed _____

Heating & A/C Agreement
_____
_____
_____
_____

Sign Placement & Maintenance Agreement
_____
_____
_____

Maintenance & Janitorial Agreement
_____
_____

Concessions
Prior to the beginning lease date, the owner will make the following modifications.
_____
_____

FIGURE 3.4
Lease checklist.

and were about to open when we were informed we were not allowed to have the words "Hairstyling" or "Hair Design" or anything similar in the sign wordage. It turns out, an existing salon in the shopping center where we were locating had not been allowed to include that in its sign and therefore we weren't either. As our salon name wasn't the sort of name that automatically told what we were, we were at a distinct disadvantage, but there was little we could do about it.

Maintenance and janitorial services. Compare costs and services between the owner providing such services and independently contracting them. Have any arrangements specified in definite terms. As an example, "The walls will be painted between January and February of each year. If touch-ups need to be made in the interim, the tenant should contact the owner, who shall see that the repairs are completed within thirty days."

Concessions. Negotiate to have the owner pay for any costs incurred should improvements or modifications need to be made to the property before your opening day, covering such items as installing electrical outlets or light fixtures, painting, erecting tables or counters, or carpeting. Obtain permission to remove items such as air conditioners or water coolers, if you plan to change their locations.

Contingency clause. Ask for a contingency clause that states you will not be responsible for the terms of the lease if you do not receive your salon license within a specific amount of time. This is possible to do, believe it or not.

Ninety-day cancellation notice. Standard notification of renewal or cancellation of leases normally is sixty days. Negotiate to increase this period to ninety days to give additional time to make a wise decision about your location.

Before signing any lease, remember to have an attorney review it and be certain to get everything in writing. Verbal assurances, promises, and guarantees normally do not hold up should a dispute arise.

SERVICES AND PRODUCTS

Besides location, the services and products you plan to offer clients should be carefully considered, as well as the prices you plan to charge. You will need to determine the proper pricing schedule to ensure a profit, before you ever style your first head of hair or sell that first bottle of shampoo. Work with your accountant on this, and refer to chapter 7 for further help. One thing about setting prices—you need to understand the difference between markup and profit. When you buy an item for $1.00 and sell it for $1.43, you have a 43 percent markup. However, your gross profit margin is only 30 percent of your retail sales. This is because although $.43 is 43 percent of $1.00, it is only 30 percent of $1.43. By factoring your overhead in relation to gross sales, you can determine your breakeven point, calculating how many bottles of shampoo or conditioner you need to sell to make the equation balance. Higher sales volume, higher markup percentages, lower overhead—all will alter this equation and result in profit or loss for the owner.

Also, your markup, and therefore your price and profit, are determined by the perceived value your product has with your clients versus the cost you pay to obtain and deliver the product or service. When assessing your competition, negotiating with suppliers, and conducting your market research, make certain you take into account the perceived value of your products and services.

It is customary in our business for the supplier and manufacturer of the various lines to strongly suggest the markup and retail price of the items you obtain from them. Do not assume you are bound by this. Perform your own study to see if that suggested retail price will tender you a sufficient profit for the operation you have.

Before you can determine what to charge in order to provide a decent profit to the salon, you must compute the unit cost of each service and product. Simply charging what is usual and customary is not sufficient as many items and services may well be under- or overpriced. If they are underpriced, especially, you need to know that if you are planning to remain in business! That is a prime reason many salons go under. They may be fully booked, all stylists working at capacity, but the salon is not returning a profit because, say, their permanent waves are priced so that the salon loses money each time that particular service is offered. When determining unit costs, which is the term we will use when defining what each particular service or product costs us to produce and market, you should employ your accountant as your partner in helping arrive at those figures.

Costs

Basically, several normal types of costs are involved. First are those costs we term variable, which include costs that change in proportion to business activity. As the production volume increases, these costs likewise increase; inversely, as the production volume decreases, so do these costs. Examples are retail products. If you sell a hundred cases of a certain brand of hair spray a year, you should be eligible for buying in volume to get a lower purchase cost, thereby lowering the overall cost factor.

If you increase personnel, you experience raises in the costs of electricity usage. If you pay personnel by a graduated percentage basis, based on service dollar volume per individual, your labor costs would increase or decrease by volume, depending on how you structure your scale. If you pay by salary, or salary plus bonus, these costs again will fluctuate. If you charge a rental booth fee instead, again your costs will differ.

If you increase a service activity, say double your perm production, you may then realize a savings on buying perm supplies, which, once again, may lower production costs of that service.

In short, any cost that is affected by production levels is termed a variable cost. Work with your accountant to determine all aspects of unit costs. You need a professional for this analysis, just as you would expect clients to seek professional services for their hair needs.

Fixed costs are the second part of the equation in determining unit costs. These costs may include such items as the owner's salary, rent, property taxes, insurances, and perhaps utility costs and depreciation. Fixed costs per unit fall lower as production increases, which may be confusing, and lead the manager to assume that costs are being reduced, when the truth is that fixed costs have not changed.

The third factor in assessing unit costs is semivariable costs. Labor costs, based on a graduated percentage pay scale, may fall into this category, or they may be better included in the variable cost category. Your accountant will help make this determination. Other examples of semivariable costs are sporadic buying opportunities such as at trade shows when product deals are offered. Another semivariable cost might be incurred if you are on a system with your telephone service whereby you pay a flat service charge, but pay an additional unit charge for calls made. At our salon we provide a toll-free number for our out-of-state clients' convenience, the cost of which fluctuates monthly, depending on usage. Again, this is a semivariable cost.

As every salon's needs and goals are different, it is virtually impossible to come up with a general formula for determining unit costs without the help of a professional knowledgeable about your particular case. Use your accountant!

To attempt to set up service and product charges and prices without first determining what the cost of each service and product will be is economic suicide. Do not just set up the same prices as your old salon, or even comparable salons in your market. Prices are not just numbers to be tossed out. Many salons go belly up because they don't set their prices properly. Thorough planning will ensure proper pricing. Your accountant will want detailed information and figures on a variety of categories, and you should be prepared to furnish these. Some costs will be hard to predict, especially without a track record or history to go by, but estimate to the best of your experience, and, as time progresses, readjust the cost figures until they are as accurate as possible.

Much of the information you will need to gauge these costs is already included in your business plan (see chapter 2). If you are determined to assess your own costs without the aid of an accountant, the book recommended in that chapter, *How to Write a Business Plan*, from the American Management Association (see Appendix B for address) will be invaluable, as will perhaps another of the AMA's publications, *How to Prepare an Effective Business Plan, A Step-by-Step Approach*. If you are fairly financially astute, you should be able to estimate unit costs with the aid of either of these references.

A personal example of the value of estimating unit costs occurred years ago in a salon I owned in the Midwest. I opened the salon with great success, working by myself, and enjoyed a full booking immediately, which was gratifying since I didn't personally know a single person in the town the day I opened. For those interested in how I achieved a full booking, the story is included in my book *You and Your Clients: Milady's Human Relations for Cosmetology* (see Appendix B for how to order).

At any rate, business prospered, things were good, and I needed another stylist almost immediately. My figures showed I was losing an average of $500 per week in business I could not physically handle and was forced to turn away. I was booked six to eight weeks in advance.

I hired a stylist, who came to me without a clientele, and in his first week, strictly from the overflow, he netted more income than he'd ever grossed in total service dollars *before* being paid his percentage. That was good for him, but there turned out to be a problem. Although I suffered no reduction in the amount of money I was grossing each week, and indeed it went up significantly, I suddenly wasn't putting money into my savings account like I had been. That puzzled me, until my accountant examined my books and discovered that with the percentage I was paying my new stylist (the average commission for the time), I was losing fifty cents every time he touched a head of hair!

My being forced to lower his percentage led him to leave me and open his own salon, even though with the new, profitable percentage he still made more than twice as much as he had at his other salon. The lesson to be had is that you can be fully booked until the year 2000 and be losing money if your prices and pay scales aren't set correctly.

An important factor to consider when determining where to open your salon is the kind of salon you want to have. Salons that are successful on purpose, and not by fortuitous accident, generally identify a particular segment of the market and aggressively go after their share of that segment. Salons that try to be "something to everybody" often end up being "nothing to nobody," which may be poor grammar, but an effective description.

If, for instance, you desire an upscale clientele but hate the thought of losing the possible income budget-conscious clients have to offer, you may discover that the two kinds of clients are very uncomfortable with each other, and you stand a good chance of attracting neither. There are ways to attract a very diverse client mix, but it is usually more effective to identify a particular clientele and pursue that group. You will pick up members from outside the targeted segment as well, but to plan the salon operation and personality around all segments is a foolhardy strategy. Opposites don't really mix, contrary to folk wisdom.

A common misconception is to think that a large number of clients is better than a few, but this may not be the case. You may be more profitable by pricing products and services high and serving those who seek a higher perceived value. Or, you may be better off doing the opposite. Whichever you do, you should know the breakeven point needed in order to survive.

You may need to obtain financing. Conventional lenders will need to know such things as:

- What are the objectives of the salon?
- How much capital will be needed for the first year and a half?
- How will the capital be used?
- How will they be paid back?
- What is your equity?
- Will you have other investors, and for how much?
- What is your track record in the past?
- What are to be the significant milestones for the salon?
- What is the debt level of the salon now?

- Who are the owners to be?
- What are the qualifications of owners and key employees?
- What are the possible liabilities?
- Are there any lawsuits or tax problems?
- What events and situations could affect the business?

Probably no investor will consider your salon unless you are planning to invest your own capital. This is easy to understand. If you do not believe in your business enough to invest your own money in it, why should anyone else?

If you apply to a bank or other institution for a loan and are turned down, a good loan officer should explain what you must do in order to qualify, so that eventually you can secure the necessary funds. Always ask what you need to do next to gain their confidence in lending you money.

Once you have secured the financing, you need to review where you are before proceeding:

- Do you have enough funds in the bank to take care of business and personal financial needs?
- Has financing been secured at the level required?
- Are your personnel needs satisfied?
- Have you determined how to structure the business, whether proprietorship, partnership, or corporation?
- Have your breakeven points been calculated?
- Have you developed the location criteria checklist?
- Do you have the necessary skills for the undertaking?
- Is your marketing plan solid, and how will you evaluate whether it is working?
- Do you have gross sales goals, pricing, and inventory management plans in place?

Here is another checklist you might use before opening the doors:

- All licenses secured.
- Business name and legal structure finalized.
- Location determined and secured.
- Lease favorable to your needs negotiated with the help of your attorney.

- Insurances taken care of.
- Advertising and marketing plans in place.
- Business cards, scheduling books, and other such operational materials on hand.
- Recordkeeping systems set up.
- Financial performance statements projected for at least three years.
- Cash flow calculated for three years.
- Vendors and suppliers chosen.
- Orders for initial inventory placed.
- Equipment and supplies contracted for.
- Staff selected.
- Special promotions planned.
- Client satisfaction standards developed.
- Inspections performed.

As soon as you begin servicing clients, you should be conducting evaluations and providing the material for future research, by finding out:

- How do new clients find out about you?
- Where do they live?
- What do they like about the salon and service or product?
- How could you improve (in their eyes)?
- Will they patronize you again?
- How do you stack up against the competition?
- What is the average sale amount?

A good concept to keep in mind is that the clients we see in our salons are not buying services or products. They are buying benefits. Learn to use the concept of features, advantages, and benefits. Most people, salon owners included, are motivated to purchase a service or product by one or more of five basic desires.

1. To be successful and achieve goals.
2. To be safe, secure, and comfortable.
3. To be appreciated, accepted, and to belong.
4. To use money and resources wisely.
5. To gain satisfaction.

Each salon service and product should be perceived by the customer as achieving at least one of these needs.

One more thing—a famous New England businessman once said that there were two rules for customer satisfaction. Rule one is "the customer is always right." Rule two is "if the customer is wrong, see rule one." By teaching your stylists and other personnel that the client is the reason they are there and able to earn a living, you can help create an attitude that will greatly lessen the number of client complaints.

The first year you own your salon will almost always be the most difficult in some ways and the most rewarding in others. Eighteen-hour days are common, when you find you begin the day as the bookkeeper and end it as the clean-up person!

Cash flow will be one of the biggest problems you face. If this is on the tight side, your projections may have to be adjusted weekly. Cash flow figures will help you identify which areas of the business require medical aid.

You will need to report your progress to your investors at regular intervals. Do not hide bad news from them, or wait until the news is overwhelming before they are advised. Doing so will, at best, make you appear incompetent as if you were ignorant or unaware of the problem. At worst, you could be perceived as perpetuating a fraud. Honest communication of a problem shows you to be a knowledgeable business person who keeps track of your business and will allow those best able to help an opportunity to come up with solutions.

Communicate with everyone involved with your business—your investors, your staff, and most importantly, your clients.

As you can begin to see, opening a new business is not as simple as one might anticipate, at least if that business is to stand a decent chance of succeeding. Then again, it is not that formidable a task when one is armed with the proper information and conducts sound planning. The days of building a clientele and then going down the street and renting a space and becoming a salon owner are probably over. It is a competitive market we find ourselves in, and likely to become even more so in the future. Only those armed with proven business practices are likely to succeed in the coming years. By taking the time to study this book and other resources, you are placing yourself in the group that will make it. This is only the first step down the road to prosperity, but be assured you are on the right path.

You are on the threshold of an exciting venture. Do it the right way and your chance of survival and success beyond your wildest dreams is within your grasp.

Good luck!

REVIEW

Before deciding to open a salon, conduct an honest self-assessment, asking yourself questions that should reveal whether you are truly prepared to own your own business. Seek information about running a small business in as many places as you can. Answer some basic questions about your market before you finalize your plans, whether you are buying an existing salon or opening a new one.

Location can determine your salon's success or failure. When deciding on a location, begin with assessing your competition. When looking at particular sites, take a Site Assessment Form to help you gather the information you need to select a good location and negotiate your lease. Services and products, along with a pricing schedule, should be determined before you actually perform any services or sell any products.

PERSONNEL

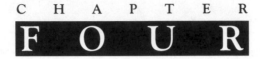

C H A P T E R

FOUR

No area is more crucial to salon success than the proper selection and development of your staff. The right people in the right positions will contribute positively to the bottom line more than any other single factor. Conversely, the right people in the wrong positions can lead to a high turnover rate that will cost you your reputation and dollars.

You must be able to define company goals, both short and long term, via the instrument of your business plan. From that, formulate a plan of action and communicate it clearly to your staff. Part of your strategy must also include motivational tactics that will ensure that the people working for you implement the business plan.

Make no mistake about this: Your salon is only as strong as its weakest link—the people you hire and supervise are your most important allies in achieving success. To develop personnel thoroughly, you must achieve the following:

- Hire the right people for the opening.
- Develop a job description and salon manual so that each employee knows exactly what is expected.
- Help employees set personal goals that are within the framework of the salon goals, and then give them the wherewithal to achieve those goals.

- Provide thorough training.
- Provide continual education.
- Motivate by personal example and leadership.
- Eliminate morale problems before they get out of hand.
- Coordinate salon activities and staff responsibilities so they are fair, impartial, and according to merit.
- Have a heart! Exhibit to your employees that you truly care about them, that they are not just the means to your financial ends, and that you have a desire for them to become the best professionals they can be.

As the owner, you are the one who sets the tone for the salon's atmosphere and ambiance. Every client who walks through the door will obtain a sense of the place, and that can be either a positive or a negative feeling, depending on you. That atmosphere is achieved either by mission or omission—make your atmosphere a result of mission! Work at cultivating a friendly, professional environment, and enlist your staff's aid in doing so, explaining what it is you are after and how it may be best obtained. Ask for suggestions—nothing motivates another person more than appealing to his or her ego, and there is nothing wrong in this.

It is tempting at times to let down your hair and become "one of the boys or girls," but it is more important to retain a certain amount of professional distance between employer and employee. This is not to say you cannot be friendly—indeed, you should take great pains to be so—but there should be clearly defined parameters that neither you nor those employed by you may cross, much as there exist parameters between parent and child. This is true in any professional relationship, and if these parameters break down, or never existed, there will probably be problems.

RECRUITING

There are many methods of obtaining qualified personnel. (Figure 4.1) Classified advertisements in local newspapers are one method. To attract the kind of talented applicant you desire for your salon, word the ad carefully. Here is a good example of such an ad that you can use for a model in writing your own.

HAIR DESIGNER
IF YOU ARE SELF-MOTIVATED, WITH THE DESIRE AND
ABILITY TO PROVIDE YOUR CLIENTS THE BEST POSSIBLE
SERVICE AND THE DESIRE TO BE AT THE TOP OF YOUR
PROFESSION, WE ARE NOT CONCERNED AT THIS POINT WITH
YOUR LACK OF EXPERIENCE. BOLD STROKES HAIR
DESIGNERS HAS A COMPREHENSIVE TRAINING PROGRAM FOR
THOSE WHO ARE SELF-STARTERS AND WISH TO ASSOCIATE
THEMSELVES WITH A WINNER. CALL [insert number] TO
ARRANGE AN INTERVIEW.

When the phone begins ringing in response to your ad, have your salon coordinator or receptionist or whoever answers your phone do the following:

- Get as much information as possible about the applicant (professional and general education, special skills, experience, etc.),

FIGURE 4.1
Sample recruitment poster.

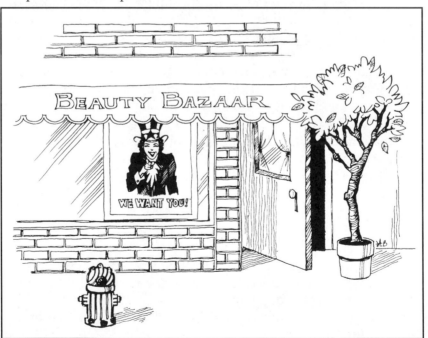

making notes not only on their answers but also on their communications skills, phone voice, and general personality. (Figures 4.2 and 4.3)

- Don't give applicants any details about the job over the phone. If they fit the profile you are looking for, tell them you would prefer to set up a formal interview where you can answer any of their questions face to face.
- Take copious notes as you talk. First impressions are important—those are the impressions all of his or her clients will have.

FIGURE 4.2
When a job applicant phones, make detailed notes recording your impressions of how pleasant and professional he or she comes across on the phone.

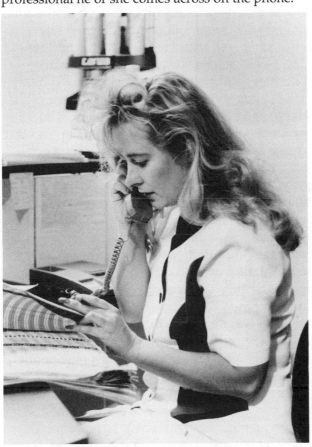

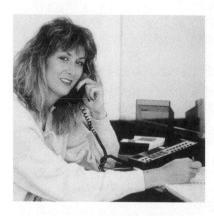

FIGURE 4.3
Listen and rate applicant's phone voice and skills.

Another avenue is to visit the cosmetology schools in your area and introduce yourself to the owners, instructors, and students themselves, if possible. Volunteer your time and talent to teach any area in which you have a special expertise. The more you can familiarize yourself with a school and its students, the better able you become at selecting graduates that would fit your salon, and the school administrators will become very willing to refer their top students to you.

Another source of cosmetologists is from other salons. This can be tricky, since it is considered bad ethics to attempt to "steal" another salon's star cutter or colorist, and usually it is bad business as well. What can you offer a top stylist except perhaps a higher percentage, and if you do that, what happens to the mood of the other stylists already on board once they find out? And, believe me, they *will* find out! If, on the other hand, you know for a reasonable fact that a stylist in another salon is unhappy with the situation, there is a way to approach this person. First, you might approach the salon owner and ask if you may talk to the stylist—this will probably obtain a reaction sort of like the one the captain of the *Titanic* gave his first mate when he told him what the loud noise was all about! But, at least you have conducted yourself ethically, and you may be surprised—the owner may agree. In which case, caveat emptor! That prize stylist may not be such a catch after all.

In general, raiding other salons for their stylists is a poor means of staffing. If, however, a stylist from another salon answers an ad, or just pops in to check the waters, by all means talk to him or her. There is nothing wrong here—you didn't initiate the query, and no one can blame others for trying to better themselves with a different job.

Sometimes it pays to advertise in the professional trades such as *American Salon*. And sometimes it pays to run ads in the school trade magazines, such as *Beauty Education,* which goes to almost all the cosmetology school owners in the country. You may have a salon in North Dakota, for instance, and a school in Maryland may have a student looking for a job in your state, and in this way a connection might be made. Stranger things have happened! I've been sort of a vagabond myself during my career, which is one of the things I love about this business—being able to relocate anywhere and get a good job in a good salon—and many times I've checked such publications' want ads for salon openings in the state I next wanted to work/play in.

The very best way to get quality applicants is to develop a good reputation. Good salons have no shortage of applicants. Sometimes, it almost seems necessary to hire a personnel manager just to screen all the applicants who seem to arrive daily in such salons. When you first open your doors, of course, you haven't yet earned that kind of reputation, but as time goes on, provided you do the things required to obtain a good repute, you will find your hiring headaches begin to diminish. It becomes analogous to colleges recruiting football players. Notre Dame, for example, has the problem of who to turn down for a football scholarship, more than it does in trying to entice blue chippers. Reputation. You don't buy it; you earn it, and once you have it, good things happen.

Once the phone begins to ring with hopefuls, and you've set up appointments, the interviewing process begins.

INTERVIEWS

Most businesses don't rush headlong into hiring people. It takes time to see if a proper fit can be achieved. Our industry has traditionally made many mistakes in this area. We need someone; so we run an ad on Friday; we interview on Monday; on Tuesday the first or second applicant is behind a chair; and by Friday night the owner has red eyes from the sleepless nights occasioned by the hairdresser from Hell who has descended upon the once peaceful salon and is threatening to send the entire business into bankruptcy by driving all the clients away.

Take your time. Insist on a minimum of at least two interviews, and probably three, before you make any decision. For those who just have to know immediately, tell them you're sorry, but such a decision cannot be made hastily, and if they are in such a hurry, perhaps yours is not the place for them to be. You will have to live by your decision, and, with today's laws, the wrong hiring decision can be not only embarrassing but costly.

First Interview

You will want to ascertain certain things about the applicant. These are some of the assessments you should be aware of:

- Know the exact job you are trying to fill and its duties and description. "Hair designer" is too vague—does the new employee have to be able to perform sophisticated perm wraps, for example? Will the employee be expected to sweep up for others or shampoo the clients? Is the person allowed to ring up purchases? What familiarity should the applicant have with certain product lines? And so on and so on. Know exactly what it is you are looking for.
- Always ask open-ended questions that avoid simple yes or no answers. Make the applicant have to think and come up with viable answers. You need an intelligent stylist, not a robot.
- Watch body language and listen carefully to what the candidate says and doesn't say, and make notes, notes, notes!
- To determine training and education, ask questions like:

  1. What cosmetology school did you attend, and when?
  2. Why did you choose this profession?
  3. Have you had classes since graduation?
  4. What were your responsibilities at your last two jobs?
  5. What part of hairdressing excites you the most and why?
  6. What were your favorite and least favorite managers like?
  7. Why did you leave your last job?
  8. Why are there lapses of time between jobs (if there are)?

- To determine an applicant's goals and work habits, ask:

  1. Why do you want to work for Bold Strokes Hair Designers?
  2. What can we expect to gain from hiring you?
  3. How do you define success?
  4. What are your earning goals? In one year? Two? Five years from now? Do you want to own your own salon?

5. What do you define as the qualities of a good leader or manager?

6. What are you looking for in us?

Once you are convinced the interviewee is qualified, ask the applicant to fill out the application form. Tell the applicant you are interviewing others and will be setting up practical tests or additional interviews with the best candidates, and you will inform people within five working days whether they will be included further in the interviewing process.

As soon as the session is over and the applicant has departed, record your impressions. You can use the form provided, or come up with one of your own. It is important you do this right away while your impressions are still fresh in your mind. It will also help you see areas you may have neglected in the interview. Sometimes we become involved in conversation and overlook significant questions.

Second Interview

Before the second interview, check out the applicant's references. Many salons ask for references and never bother to use them. Use them! They are a highly valuable index to the applicant's abilities, skills, and attitudes.

When verifying information from references and getting their opinions, identify yourself and the purpose of your call. Don't under any circumstance give the applicant's name to anyone but the person

BOLD STROKES HAIR DESIGNERS
INTERVIEW IMPRESSIONS

Grooming/Wardrobe _____

Communication (phone and interview)_____

   Ability to listen _____

   Articulation _____

   Responsiveness _____

   Answering ability (quick, attentive?) _____

   Modulation of voice_____

Personality (use one word that best describes)_____

Additional comments (good or poor) _____

_____

furnishing you the reference information. If the person listed is no longer with the company or is in a different position, try to find that person.

If anyone is suspicious of who you are and why you are phoning, request the person call you back after verifying your phone number in the phone book. If the reference will not give you information, ask to speak to a superior, as others higher up often have a better understanding of your need for this information.

If you obtain sufficient verbal information, there is no need to request written data. Make good notes, and keep all such records for two years. By law, you must furnish the candidate with reference information if it is requested within two years of the reference check. Even though the candidate's request must be made in writing, you are required to give only a verbal response.

If information received contradicts what the applicant has told you, inform him or her. It is only courteous to give the applicant the opportunity to correct what may be an error in the reference's files.

When you phone the reference, ask this sample list of questions:

1. Position candidate held, title, dates of employment.
2. What were the responsibilities with the company?
3. How would you rate the applicant's performance? Why do you say that?
4. How was attendance and punctuality?
5. How did he or she get along with coworkers? Superiors?
6. What were strengths? Weaknesses?
7. What particular duty is the applicant best in? What needs work?
8. Why did the applicant leave? Would you rehire him or her? Why or why not?
9. Is there anything else that could help my evaluation?

If everything checks out satisfactorily, it is time to bring in the applicant for a second interview. During this interview, you should

- Ask most of the same questions so that you can determine if answers are consistent and perhaps reveal additional information.
- Look for "red flags" you may have missed in the first interview, such as nervousness, immaturity, or personal problems.
- Have the applicant complete any practical exams, such as performing a haircut or perm wrap, that you require.

If the person seems to fit so far, schedule the third interview.

Third Interview

This is the interview where you sell yourself to the candidate. Go over the job description again and ask how the applicant feels about it. State specific expectations. Then make an offer. Have a formal letter prepared, outlining compensation, benefits, and any probationary periods. If you require a no-competition agreement, this is the time to have it signed. The candidate should have been made aware of such a requirement at the first interview.

Welcome the person to the team and introduce your staff! You have both just completed an arduous but worthwhile process, and you have probably made a better fit for your salon than most of your competitors. With this process, your newest employee knows that you value his or her position highly—why else would you take so much trouble in finding the right person for it?

LEGAL ASPECTS OF INTERVIEWING

There are some things that by law you are not allowed to ask an applicant. These are the individual's sex, birthplace, religion, race, or primary language. If the candidate offers any of this information or attaches a photograph, it is best to eliminate it, because of possible legal implications. You must base your hiring decision solely on skills and none of these factors.

On the other hand, you are allowed to ask candidates for their name, place of residence, educational background, military experience, work experience, membership in organizations, references, and the name, address, and phone number of persons to call in the event of an emergency.

WHEN A STAFF MEMBER LEAVES

Sadly, there will come times when some of your staff may leave for personal or professional reasons. If a stylist who has been generally unproductive or negative resigns, let the person go! If, on the other hand, a talented, productive, cohesive part of your staff wants to leave, make every effort possible to identify and work out the problem.

There are three valid reasons to terminate an employee:

1. The employee won't do the job.
2. The employee can't do the job.
3. The employee is negative and spreads the disease throughout the salon.

If you have such an individual, especially in a small salon of, say, four people, you have no logical choice but to let that person go. One ineffective staff member may cost you 25 percent of your productivity. It is a good idea, if you can, to have the departing employee sign a voluntary resignation letter, which may protect you from unemployment benefits claims. Here is an example of such a letter:

I, _____ , hereby submit my

voluntary resignation, effective as of _____

I am resigning because

_____ I have obtained another position.

_____ I am relocating.

_____ I am entering a new field.

_____ I feel I am unsuited for my present position.

_____ I wish to increase my income.

_____ Other. _____

| _____ | _____ |
| Date | Employee Signature |

Immediately ask the employee to remove personal items and tools from the workplace. Arrange for the employee to receive a final paycheck. Cancel all benefits and advise about any conversion privileges, such as insurances. Conduct an exit interview to learn how to keep good employees. (If the person is averse to this, ask for a letter detailing what you could have done to avoid the situation.) Try to have the employee leave on as good terms as possible.

In many salons, when a stylist or designer leaves or is discharged, the salon coordinator or receptionist is directed to tell all those phoning in for that person's services that the stylist is no longer with the company, and they don't have a forwarding address. This is unprofessional and not worthy of a quality salon. Instead, isn't it better to tell the caller you are sorry Lynn is no longer with the salon but you are sure that the caller would be happy if you could book him or her with Peggy? If the person still asks for Lynn's new location, pass it on if you know it. We try to go a step further at our salon, volunteering the information before the client can ask, and even cheerfully giving the client the phone number, although we do invite the client back to our salon with another designer.

Do not allow discharged employees to retain keys or methods of entry into the salon, or access to any records, client files, or information of that sort. Those are the property of the salon. It is a good idea to inform new stylists of this policy when hiring them.

The best defense against having to fire employees is to make sure you get the right ones to begin with! Use the methods outlined in this chapter, and your discharge rate will drastically decline.

MOTIVATING STAFF

The twelve most important considerations an employer should offer to motivate staff, according to the *Business Owner's Handbook* and determined by a survey of employees, are:

1. challenging work.
2. two-way communication.
3. recognition.
4. pay equal to performance.
5. company pride.
6. fairness.
7. autonomy.
8. clear performance goals.
9. training.
10. harmonious environment.
11. job security.
12. benefit package.

RECORD-KEEPING

All employee work records must be kept for seven years. Other employee and business records must be kept as per the list below, as furnished by the *Business Owner's Handbook.*

Item/Document	Retention Period
Accident reports/claims (settled cases)	7 yrs.
Accts. payable/Accts. receivable/Notes receivable ledgers & schedules	7 yrs.
Audit reports	Permanently
Bank reconciliations/statements	7 yrs./3 yrs.
Capital stock and bond records: ledgers transfer registers, stubs showing issues, record of interest coupons, opinions, etc.	Permanently
Cash books	Permanently
Charts of accounts/Journals	Permanently
Checks (canceled—see exception below)	7 yrs.
Checks (canceled for important payments, e.g., taxes, property purchases, special contracts, etc. Checks should be filed with the papers pertaining to the underlying transaction.)	Permanently
Contracts, mortgages, notes, and leases expired/ still in effect	7 yrs./Permanently
Correspondence general/legal & important matters	2 yrs./Permanently
Deeds, mortgages, and bills of sale	Permanently
Duplicate deposit slips	2 yrs.
Employment applications	3 yrs.
Expense analysis/expense distribution schedules	7 yrs.
Financial statements (year-end)	Permanently
Garnishments	7 yrs.
General/private ledgers, year-end trial balance	Permanently
Insurance policies expired/current—reports, claims, policies, etc.	3 yrs./Permanently
Internal audits & reports	3 yrs.
Inventories of products, materials & supplies/ Physical inventory tags	7 yrs.
Invoices (to customers, from vendors)	7 yrs.
Magnetic tape & tab cards	1 year
Minute books of directors, stockholders, bylaws, & charter	Permanently
Option records (expired)	7 yrs.
Patents & related papers/Trademark registrations & copyrights	Permanently

Payroll records/Time books & cards/Personnel files (terminated)	7 yrs.
Petty cash vouchers	3 yrs.
Plant cost ledgers	7 yrs.
Property appraisals done by outside appraisers	Permanently
Property records, including costs, depreciation reserves, year-end trial balances, depreciation schedules, blueprints, and plans	Permanently
Purchase orders (except purchasing dept. copy)	1 year
Receiving sheets	1 year
Retirement & pension records	Permanently
Requisitions	1 year
Sales commission reports	3 yrs.
Scrap & salvage record (inventories, sales, etc.)	7 yrs.
Stenographers' notebooks	7 yrs.
Stock & bond certificates (canceled)	7 yrs.
Stockroom withdrawal forms	1 year
Subsidiary ledgers	7 yrs.
Tax returns & work sheets, revenue agents' reports, & other documents relating to determination of tax liability	Permanently
Training manuals	Permanently
Union agreements	Permanently
Voucher register & schedules	7 yrs.
Vouchers for pymts. to vendors, employees, etc.	7 yrs.
Withholding tax statements	7 yrs.

Before you put out your first ad for hiring a stylist, certain legal requirements must be met. The ones covered here are federal. You may have additional legal responsibilities in your particular state, and your city or county or parish may have additional requirements, so check with the proper authorities before you begin your hiring process. If you are unclear about what authority you need to consult, ask either your attorney or the state (or whatever governmental entity you plan to open the business within) business licensing agency, as well as the local branch of the Internal Revenue Service.

To satisfy federal law, you must have a federal employer identification number for starters. Check Circular E from the Internal Revenue Service, which explains such things as withholding federal taxes, social security taxes, and payments. New employees must fill out federal Form W-4 that shows their withholding exemptions and social security number. OSHA requirements must also be adhered to, and there are certain recent changes you should be aware of, obtainable by writing to the Occupational Safety and Health Administration, U.S. Department of Labor, 200 Constitution Avenue NW, Washington, DC, 20210, or phoning (202) 523-8151. Clients must be informed of any and all chemicals in any of your preparations or items for sale, and their properties. This must be posted, so check with OSHA as to the exact requirements. In the future, there may be severe penalties for noncompliance, and, like speeding on the highway, ignorance of the law is not an allowed defense.

Also, employees will probably have to be covered by workers' compensation and both federal (FUTA) and state unemployment taxes. Your liability as an employer begins the minute the employee is hired. If you decide to provide certain benefits, such as health insurances or pension or profit-sharing programs, you must be in accordance with the Employee Retirement Income Security Act (ERISA), which has two kinds of requirements, disclosure to employees and reporting to government agencies.

Can you begin to see why all books such as this urge new business owners to retain the services of such professionals as an attorney and an accountant! It becomes a bit more complicated than when you were eleven and opened your first lemonade stand. But most of these laws are in place to protect you and your employees, as well as the public you serve. Don't despair. It may all seem a bit overwhelming, but it's really not—once you begin it will become easier than it first appears. Of course, it doesn't hurt to have a competent advisor to help you through what may seem a veritable maze of papers, permits, and red tape. Aid is readily available, too. See Appendix A for a complete list of agencies and helpful establishments that are there to serve you for either no charge at all or a very nominal fee, in most instances, in all phases of starting up and running your business.

Other agencies you should be aware of regarding their requirements and your legal responsibilities as an employer are the U.S. Equal Employment Opportunity Commission (EEOC), whose address is EEOC, 2401 E Street NW, Washington, DC, 20507, (800) USA-EEOC. Phone or write them if you have any questions or need information about civil rights or employment discrimination.

You cannot hire illegal aliens, but the law forbids discrimination in hiring based on appearance, language, or surname. Each employee, regardless of national origin, is required to complete U.S. Form I-9, which verifies citizenship or legal alien status, as per the Immigration Reform and Control Act of 1986.

Other programs exist for armed forces veterans. For details contact the Veterans' Employment and Training Service, Office of the Assistant Secretary for Veterans' Employment and Training, 200 Constitution Avenue NW, Room S1316, Washington, DC, 20210, (202) 523-9110. There are state and local branches as well. Consult your local phone directory or ask the operator for assistance in locating them.

There are various minority and women's programs and agencies listed in Appendix A that you may want to check into. Many have programs that are of benefit to employers hiring personnel from these categories. As each state is different and some have more such agencies and commissions than others, please check with your own local authorities for more information.

ALTERNATIVES TO HIRING

For certain of your general skilled employees, such as receptionists, salon coordinators, and bookkeepers, you may want to consider a leasing arrangement, rather than hiring them yourself. Leasing from a personnel management business gives you a permanent employee, and one of the chief advantages is in insurances and benefits—not to mention that the management firm will do a professional job in screening candidates.

Another option is in hiring independent contractors or renting workstation space. If you do so, be very certain you abide by the IRS's definition of such a self-employed person. Generally, the requirements will not be met if you pay these employees by the hour or day, require them to wear any kind of uniform, furnish them with tools or equipment, or if you insist they be under your direct, ongoing supervision. If you fail in any of these areas, no matter what your agreement, the IRS can impose severe penalties. In general, I personally do not like such arrangements as booth rentals, but this is purely a personal observation. You may find the arrangement very beneficial. My own feeling is that usually professionalism is sacrificed, and it is very difficult to maintain the kind of quality desired in such arrangements. There are exceptions, however, as in anything, and staffing with self-employed personnel may be ideal for your situation and work very well. Just be certain you are in complete compliance with tax laws, as the IRS is very strict about proper compliance and reporting.

Finally, remember above all else that we are primarily a service business. As such, we are labor intensive and rely heavily upon our staff to create income and establish the salon's reputation. Taking care to provide top-quality staff members should be the owner's very highest priority. If, after all your precautions and careful hiring practices you end up with a negative employee, try to resolve the situation immediately, by all means possible. But if all efforts fail, no matter how much income that person may bring to the salon, it is usually in the best interests of the business to terminate such an employee, and this action should not be postponed, but effected immediately. If, as we stated earlier, you have four people working for you and one is spreading a negative atmosphere, you have 25 percent of your workforce affecting productivity and the disease will usually spread. So, exercise it! Tough words, but necessary. (Figure 4.4)

FIGURE 4.4
One negative, gossipy stylist can really disrupt business.

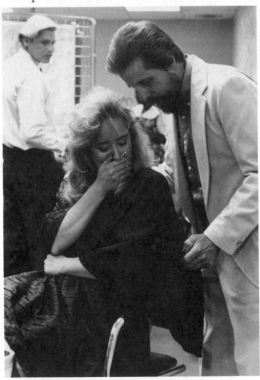

Let's hope, however, that with the aid of this book and your own good sense and knowledge, such action will seldom become necessary.

The surest way to avoid negativism within the salon environment is simply this: hire smart!

REVIEW

Nothing is more crucial to salon success than the proper selection and development of staff. The best way to attract quality applicants is to develop a good reputation. The interviewing process should include at least two interviews, and three is better. Besides following federal regulations for hiring, find out what additional legal requirements are mandated by your state, city, or county.

Sometimes, even when you are careful about hiring, it becomes necessary to terminate an employee. If you find an employee acting in a negative way, try to resolve the situation. But if all efforts fail, it is usually in the best interest of the salon to terminate the employee.

TRAINING

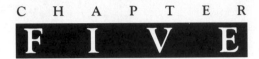

C H A P T E R
FIVE

As our business is a labor-intensive type, it follows that a great deal of care and thought be invested in creating a training program for salon personnel that will create and maintain the proper level of quality necessary to achieve salon goals. A salon owner can have all the lofty plans in the world, but unless he or she has the personnel who can implement those plans, they can only fail.

"But education is expensive!" you say, and you are right. However, *not* educating your staff will prove to be even more expensive!

Let us accept that education and training are necessary to the health and success of the salon. Are there methods of achieving a training program that won't necessarily cost the salon owner an arm and a leg? Of course there are!

This may be a good time to take a look at some of the more traditional means of achieving such training, and perhaps we will see that there are fresher ways of educating ourselves and our staffs that we previously hadn't considered.

TRADE SHOWS

In the past, many of us thought that the best means of attaining new knowledge in the field was to attend the many trade shows that are normally sponsored by product companies in conjunction with their distributors. This remains a very valuable source of new ideas and techniques, but it may no longer be the best educational source available. With the technology explosion we do not have to wait for new ideas to be filtered down to us via the trade shows. If something fashion-wise happens in Paris or London or Barcelona on Monday, we can literally know of it by the following week at the latest, and, in some instances, the very next day.

How? Very simply—by the miracle of videotape.

Videotapes can deliver new and vitally necessary information in our field much quicker, and can be played over and over in the privacy and comfort of our living rooms. We can even zoom in for a closeup of the artist's hands as well as play back complicated or intricate techniques until we thoroughly understand and master them—a far cry from the days when we had to sit eighteen rows back in a packed auditorium and try to pick up what was being done on a stage a mile and a half away, not to mention having to struggle to hear what was being disseminated over the buzz of the conversations on all four sides.

This does not mean that trade shows are outdated or a total waste of your time, money, and energy. They are still, and always will be, highly valuable for observing fashion and new techniques for achieving that fashion, and for the social networking that is important to our self-assurance as stylists. However, we are no longer dependent solely upon them for the latest in knowledge.

And, for most trade shows, it should prove profitable for a salon to develop an attendance strategy that will allow personnel to glean more from live shows than before. One such strategy might be to send only one stylist to the show. He or she could then conduct a seminar on what was observed and learned at the show for the rest of the stylists. Say you have four stylists on board in your salon. You could send each stylist to a different trade show and get four times as much education value for the salon for the same price as sending all the stylists to the same show. At a large show, with many different exhibitors and workshops, you could do the same. Send each stylist to a different educational event, then have the stylist who attended each show pass on the information and knowledge learned. Clearly, this is a more efficient and cost-productive method than sending all the stylists to the same show and/or workshop.

Another benefit can be gained with this method. Having stylists impart what they have seen and learned forces them to be more observant, knowing they will be expected to relay what they have learned to their fellow stylists. Better notes are taken, and the level of education being brought back to the salon improves, as does the individual stylist's powers of observation and retention, helping produce and mold a more highly qualified professional.

The general business world operates this way. In a successful corporation, employees, managers, technical workers, and salespeople are sent to a variety of educational experiences—seminars, workshops, lectures—and are expected to bring back the knowledge gained and pass it on to others in the company. A major corporation wouldn't dream of sending every single person in a specific department to a work-related workshop. They would send one or two key individuals, and those representatives would then bring back the training for the rest of the department. This is just effecting sound business practices in your training program, practices common to business in general and highly successful businesses in particular, and stretching your education dollar.

If each show or workshop were to cost $100, sending four stylists to the same workshop is only duplicating the same effort, giving back to the salon only $100 worth of educational value at four times the monetary outlay. On the other hand, sending four stylists to four different workshops will return to the salon $400 worth of additional education. Not only does the salon profit with such an arrangement, but so do the individual stylists, for now they are exposed to three other shows and the education those additional shows provided. It's a win-win situation for everyone.

VIDEOTAPES

Where you are located geographically may have an impact on what videotapes are available to you. One of the advantages I have had in working in many parts of the country is learning that what is available to a particular area is not equal nationwide. Without naming parts of the country, I have been in areas where there were over eight hundred videotapes available to the local stylists, and I have been in other areas where not even twenty could be located.

The problem is, most training videos as well as most other educational opportunities come to us via the supply companies we deal with. And, some suppliers have found their comfort levels and have chosen not to make available to their customers all that is possible. It is expensive, no doubt, to stock dozens or hundreds of videotapes, and this is undoubtedly one major reason more such videos are not readily available in certain areas. Another reason is that the stylists in a particular area, for a variety of reasons, may not be asking for videos. One, they may be simply unaware that such education is attainable, and two, like the supplier, they may have found their own comfort level, and do not wish to expend the effort to keep updated on new technology and techniques.

More often, I suspect, the average stylist simply is not aware of the plethora of video education available, or does not see the immense value in this type of learning, having been developed as a stylist on trade shows and not attaching much faith to other forms of learning.

As in any industry, the learning explosion is upon us, and the old learning curve is a thing of the past. There is no such thing as a "learning curve" these days. It is an accelerated light show, full of dazzle and pop, and if we wait around for a trade show to deliver the techniques of the future, we are falling rapidly behind the innovators in the industry.

This is the way it used to work: The creative geniuses in our profession would develop their grand ideas and put together, over several months, a presentation. The sponsoring agencies, the product manufacturers, would then promote and sell tickets for these presentations, and we, the hairstyling mass, would attend these cumbersome, time-consuming affairs to gather information that was probably months, if not years, old.

Today, if you're Alexandre of Paris and you get an inspiration, you make a phone call or two and get a film crew together. Or you shoot it yourself with the new, lightweight, sophisticated video cameras, and presto, you have a new educational tape out available worldwide within days. No longer do you have to wait for the Spring Extravaganza Show of Shows if you're Alan Edwards or Jean Braa or any other super-talented artist. You shoot the new haircut technical today and start mailing it off tomorrow.

Don't make the mistake of believing you have to have every single tape ever made to remain current—this is not the case at all. Most of those artists producing tapes are highly talented and qualified, but, in general, videos produced follow trends, and if you acquire new tapes every month or so from major brand names, for most purposes you will remain on top of the game. Rather than concentrate all of your eggs in one educational basket, it may be wise to alternate artists from time to time, thereby obtaining different perspectives on styles and techniques.

Video clubs are available from manufacturers, the artists themselves, distributors, trade magazines, and a number of sources. Be alert to certain things, however. Sometimes a prominent artist is producing tapes and distributing them through a national salon or product chain. If you subscribe to that distributor you may believe you are obtaining the latest tapes when, in fact, the distributor is holding up the tapes so that its member salons view them first. While working at Snobs in New Orleans for Anthony Jones (one of the true innovators in our business and a transplanted Englishman) we discovered that the tapes we had been buying showing a European stylist, which were distributed in this country via a well-known product company, were often over a year old. The company had several salons of its own and gave the tapes to them first, after which they were sold to member salons nationwide and represented as the latest of that artist's work. After several months of sales to subscriber salons, the same tapes, now many months old, were then advertised in the trade journals and made available to any salon or stylist. Again, these tapes were represented as being the very latest from the star of the videos. Once this was learned, Anthony merely put in a phone call to the artist and we obtained the tapes directly from him.

The point is, all is not always as it appears. What happened here is not that unusual, and means that educational videos are not always as current as they are supposed to be. If all you mean to do is remain reasonably current, then most tapes available will be satisfactory for your purposes. If, however, you envision a salon on the "cutting edge" of fashion, then you might want to investigate further to ensure you are, indeed, receiving the very latest video education. One very good way is to simply telephone the renowned stylist, ask what the latest release is, and how you can obtain a copy of it.

On trips, vacation and business, make it a practice to stop in and visit salons and ask them where they get their education. You may find avenues you were unaware of and may also have information those salons were unaware of. Networking in this fashion is another win-win situation, since stylists in other geographical areas are not direct competitors and you can only aid and assist each other.

However you obtain your videotapes, it will prove to be one of the best eduational purchases you will ever make, and at a lower cost than the ticket to a major show. (Figure 5.1)

FIGURE 5.1
Viewing a training video with another stylist can be valuable and fun.

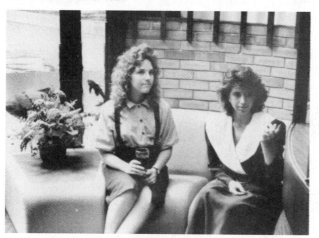

TRAINING NEEDS

When planning your educational schedule for the year, plan for *all* phases of your stylists' training. Technical information and training are important, but of equal or perhaps even more importance in today's world are training and competence in communication and sales techniques.

Traditionally, most trade shows, videos, and other forms of education have concentrated on the technical aspects of hairstyling and designing. More and more, however, workshops in communicating with clients and with each other have begun to take their place with the technical experts, and none too soon! As much of the educational dollar as is provided for technical education should probably be spent on learning communication, sales, business, and human behavior skills. The successful salon of the nineties and beyond into the next exciting century is not going to be the salon that merely knows the latest cut—it will be the salon that knows the people skills that enable it to effectively market that cut.

All the education is not through industry sources. Look to the leaders in other businesses and trades for ideas you can use in your own. Here's a good example. Several years ago, I interviewed a man who managed the outlet of a very prominent and successful national retailing chain. From that chat, I learned that retailers place larger sizes of the same product on the right of the shelf. In other words, if they have a product, say shampoo, in three sizes they place the small on the left, medium in the middle, and large on the right. The reason? More than nine out of ten people in this country are right-handed, and that means it is physically easier to pick up an object nearer that hand than the other. This man's company did a study that found that sales of larger sizes increased more than 20 percent when they placed the bottles in this manner. Immediately, we began to do the same with the retail items in our own salon, and though I cannot report the exact percentage of sales increase, it did go up significantly.

This is but one example of how to use information other business persons have available solely for the asking—especially businesses that are noncompetitive.

When you are in businesses that are obviously successful, begin observing what makes them that way. I assure you—it's no accident! Huge conglomerates spend millions upon millions to find out such pieces of information as what colors make people spend more (red is excellent in cash register areas), how to arrange sizes of the same product, or even what the best height is to display slower-moving items. If you use your head and make the acquaintance of managers of these stores, you can pick their brains and find out what they know for nothing. We all have those people as clients already—why not ask them what they know? It is a rarity when such a person won't be flattered by you asking for his or her opinion in your business.

There are also a myriad of professional and trade magazines in areas we might not have considered before, but which can have great value in our specialized business. For instance, there are dozens of trade publications on everything from retailing in general to retailing in particular (for a specific product or industry). Even though the publication may be designed for a specific industry, most of the information can be useful in almost any other business. You get the advantage of sophisticated studies for pennies!

Simple observation can be valuable. When you enter businesses you know to be successful, outline what it is you think makes that business a good one. It might be anything from the decor to the items offered to the way the sales clerk greets you. Observe and then use this information to upgrade and improve your own salon and personnel. If we use our eyes and ears, many times the answers to our problems are right there before us.

Your own staff is one of the best sources of training you'll ever have. There is not one person styling hair who doesn't know something about this business that no one else does, even if that person is but hours from cosmetology school graduation. Being human gives each of us a different perspective on everything ever learned. (Did you know that no two individuals ever see exactly the same colors when viewing an object?) To everything in life, we bring our own unique personality. This means that we may think we know what each of our stylists is capable of, but usually we are in for a surprise when we discover the reality. Ask one of your stylists to give the rest of you a class in any phase of our profession, and I will bet you a good sum of money you will be amazed at what you will learn.

And videotape your own classes! Start to build your own library of video education. How many times has a new stylist come on board and you find yourself wasting valuable time, repeating lessons taught over and over to the stylists who preceded him or her? For instance, if you have a procedure you want followed in blow-drying or air-forming hair, wouldn't it be better to have a video to let the new stylist learn from, rather than deliver the same class over and over, every time you hire someone else? Once you have taped a particular class, you free up the time you would have had to spend teaching that subject, forever. All that will be required are periodic updates, at most.

Use the resources available that are right beneath your nose! I guarantee you will not only learn something useful, but also make a staffer gain in confidence and ability, and isn't that a valuable thing? Of course!

You could also use such videos to educate your clients. Blow-drying is a good example. In our salon, Bold Strokes Hair Designers, we have a particular method we want all of our stylists to use when air-forming hair. Our method ensures the hair will be dried in a healthy state, and it also utilizes a method that is easy for the client and is adaptable to virtually any hairstyle. We prepared a video to train our stylists, and discovered our clients loved it as well, as it was an invaluable aid to learn to dry their own hair. So now we have several copies. Some are available to our stylists and some are available to our clients. Occasionally, we'll play the tape in the waiting area for new clients to view.

Another source of training that is inexpensive is networking with noncompeting salons and stylists. Make the acquaintance of stylists outside the area you draw from and offer to trade workshops and classes with them. If you have a particular expertise in an area, inform them of that, and ask if you can trade information. You'll give them a class in razor techniques in exchange for a workshop in telephone etiquette. Don't make it an opportunity to exhibit one-upmanship, but create a truly cooperative affair from which both salons benefit. You may even create a network of several salons for educational purposes. Competition is fine, but cooperation can be even more productive and profitable, for everyone involved.

Whatever training methods you use, "big-dealize" the results. Praise your stylists who attend events not only privately, but publicly. Let clients know. Tell them, "Janice just attended a workshop for vertical hair-loops." You can even run advertisements with the information, which accomplishes two things: (1) It massages the stylist—and a massaged stylist is a happy, productive stylist, and (2) it informs potential clients that yours is a salon committed to education, and therefore probably quality. You are showing you revere education, and that is impressive to discerning consumers.

Many training opportunities are also available just for the asking. Most product distributors will gladly set up product knowledge classes for you and your staff at no cost.

One word of caution that comes from personal experience. Whenever you hold education in the salon itself, keep in mind that such an event is no place for alcohol or drugs. Introducing these substances into a learning environment does nothing but harm and will render the experience useless. The salon is never the place for drugs at any time, especially not when attempting to learn something.

Another excellent, too-often-overlooked source of knowledge is available textbooks. Major trade publishers such as Milady (the publisher of the book you are now reading) have extensive lists of dozens and dozens of books, pamphlets, and other written materials that can be obtained for very reasonable costs and cover virtually every facet of the business, from the technical end to the people skills end. If you don't already have a professional library, begin to build one, starting with basic texts and adding other topics and subjects as you go. Make these books available to your stylists and insist that they review the list and read them. Every other profession that can call itself successful pays attention to the written material available for the field. Include sales texts as well and even forecast publications such as the Naisbitt *Megatrends* series, time-management and supervisory books such as the *One Minute Manager*, and motivational books and courses by Dale Carnegie and others.

Check out course offerings at local universities, community colleges, and trade schools for classes that may be profitable for you and your staff to take. Often, schools will offer reduced rates if you audit such courses rather than take them for credit.

One last word about training. There is yet another area often neglected, and that is training for the next position. If you have any designated position or title within your salon other than stylist and owner, you should be training a replacement for each position. For example, if you maintain a level system of stylists, say three levels, you should have stylists at each lower level in training to be able to move into the next level. (Figure 5.2) If you have other positions such as managers, assistant managers, salon coordinators, or receptionists, there should be persons in training to assume the next highest position. This ensures a smooth continuity in the event personnel depart, especially at the key positions. In small salons this is difficult, but in salons of four people and more, key positions should be covered, so that a qualified person can step in and perform the duties of that position should it become suddenly vacant.

FIGURE 5.2
Train a replacement for each position.

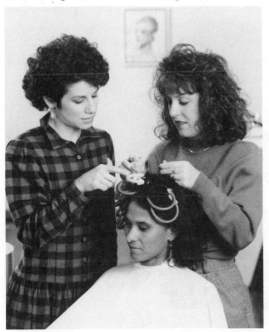

Let's say you have a position you call the "salon coordinator," and part of the job description calls for this person to maintain inventory, ordering same when needed and interfacing with salespersons. If he or she decides to leave on short or no notice, for whatever reason, you would be in a bind unless you had someone waiting in the wings who had been training for that position and could take over without the salon missing a beat—someone familiar with the ordering and inventory system. Can you see the value in having a training system in place that provides for such contingencies?

For some positions, training may consist of bringing in other resources, such as your insurance broker or your accountant or others connected with the business end of your enterprise.

Use each and every training resource you can imagine, and your salon will become the leader in its area quicker than you could have ever dreamed. Use videos, workshops, networking, colleges, other trades—use whatever applies to your business and develop a broad view when thinking of education.

In short, there are many more opportunities available for salon education than we might assume at first glance, far more than the obvious ones of trade shows. (Figure 5.3) Seek them out, use them, and watch you and your staff grow—as they grow, so will your salon!

FIGURE 5.3
Resources are essentials to further salon training and education.

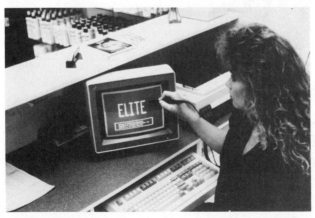

REVIEW

Ours is a service business, so care must be taken to train employees to create the proper level of quality necessary to achieve salon goals. Although trade shows remain a valuable source of new ideas and techniques, other training methods might be more cost effective and efficient. The development of videotapes has changed the industry, and new information can be passed quickly from one part of the country to another.

Technical information is important, but make sure to address other areas crucial to your success, particularly communication and sales techniques.

INVENTORY

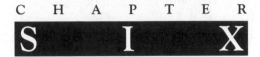

There are no unimportant parts of your business. There are parts that are more exciting than others—for instance, taking the nightly deposit to the bank can definitely be a thrill! Inventory probably ranks under those functions you would rather turn over to someone else, and if that is your choice, so be it. Take care, however, to trust your inventory control to someone reliable, as improper control of the inventory can not only harm the business, but cripple it beyond the point of a cure.

One of the first things you need to do is get a handle on how much inventory to carry. Too many of a product can eat at your profit margin; too little can result in losing sales if you don't have it readily at hand when the customer wants it. (Figure 6.1) When clients always have to wait for you to order a product, they simply look for a place that already has the item on its shelves. It is beneficial to be able to accurately forecast your inventory needs and the rates at which it depletes, as quickly as possible. Proper control procedures will help you achieve this goal.

PRICING

Again, a reminder is in order here to be certain that your prices are set properly on inventoried items (see chapter 7 for an in-depth discussion).

FIGURE 6.1
Too much of a product can eat at your profit
margin; too little can lose sales.

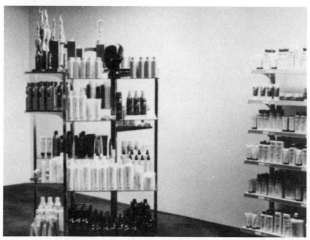

You must understand the difference between markup and profit, which
are mutually exclusive items and most definitely not the same. If you buy
a facial cleansing bar for $1.00 and sell it for $1.43, you have a 43 percent
markup, but your profit margin (and this is *gross,* not net) on the item is
only 30 percent, because though $.43 is 43 percent of $1.00, it is only 30
percent of $1.43. By figuring what your overhead is in relation to your
gross sales, you can determine your breakeven point. The breakeven in
the example cited will occur when the overhead is equal to 30 percent of
the gross sales of the item. Knowing this will enable you to calculate how
many cleansing bars you will need to sell to make the equation balance.
Lower overhead, higher sales volume, or a higher markup percentage will
each alter the equation and result in a plus or minus profit for the salon.

   Value of the product is essentially meaningless. What is important
is the perceived value the product has with your clients. If you can find a
similar product at a lower cost that has a similar perceived value with
your clientele, you can maintain your markup percentage and create a
bargain for your clients, causing profits to rise through volume. Or, you
can increase your markup percentage, in which case your volume will
probably not increase significantly, but your profits will as you have
increased your gross margin. On the other hand, if the perceived value is
lower in clients' eyes, sales may drop even if prices are lower. Always

remember: People buy perceived value, not actual value, whether you are talking retail or service sales.

Keep in mind that three factors determine the profitability of your retail sales: gross sales, gross profit margins, and overhead expenses. You can control two of these—overhead expenses and gross profit margins. You have little direct control over gross sales, being able to influence them only by your marketing efforts, so the first two factors should receive a great deal of consideration. Don't set your prices just because the distributor says this is what everyone else charges. Everyone else may be losing their shirt! If you determine there is not sufficient profit in those items, it may be time to consider implementing your own lines or finding different sources for your inventoried items.

Inventory left on the shelves or in the back room too long before it is sold can be fatal to your profitability. There is a cost involved in storing inventory or in having it on the shelf. Think about it. You pay for the space it occupies, either in the form of rent or in payment for the property and building. You pay for someone to unload it, unpack it, price it, and put it on the shelf or in the storeroom. You pay someone to dust the bottle periodically. You pay someone to ring up the sale and you probably pay a commission to the person who sold it. You pay heating and/or air conditioning costs. You perhaps pay for advertising or promotions for the item. Inventory and/or property taxes should be factored in, especially during critical times of the year. Inflation has an effect, as does the effect of the yen on the American dollar. You can literally trace dozens of factors that affect the price of a bottle of shampoo. Many costs are involved in that bottle of shampoo, and if it sits in a back room or on a shelf too long, you are losing money, perhaps significant amounts.

Deals that are available at trade shows may seem attractive, and maybe they are, but the sale price is only one part of the equation. You have to determine how soon the product will be moved or used to see if it really is that great of a deal. You may be surprised at what you discover once you understand how to figure in all the costs of a retail or for-use item. Many times it is better to pay a higher price and keep smaller amounts in stock than to take advantage of what seems to be a fantastic deal. Perhaps a better idea is to form a loose consortium of salons in your area and purchase such deals in one salon's name, and then each take a portion of the shipment, thereby obtaining goods at a cheaper price and still maintaining a lower inventory.

CHOOSING AN ACCOUNTANT

Once again, at the risk of sounding like a broken record, here is another area in which the services of a good accountant are crucial. Selecting the right accountant for your salon is the first requirement. Howard Scott, in an article in the May–June, 1992, issue of *Independent Business* (IB) *Magazine* lists seven steps to choosing an accountant for small businesses such as hairstyling salons:

1. Make certain your prospective accountant concentrates on small businesses. Many PAs and CPAs who deal mostly with individuals, large corporations, or quasi-public concerns don't have a good handle on small business concerns and problems.

2. Ask for and check out referrals from current clients, asking hard questions about how the accountant helps them run their own business more profitably and if they're satisfied with the services provided and what they have gained from the association.

3. Ask who exactly will be your accountant. You don't want to sign up with the boss and then be assigned to the summer intern!

4. Does the accountant keep abreast of tax changes? Ask about new legislation that might affect your salon. Does the firm put out a newsletter detailing these changes as part of its services?

5. Arrange to pay your accountant on an annual basis, ensuring that the fee covers all accounting work, advisory services, and your personal taxes. This way, you'll know in advance how much your accounting bill will be and can better plan your budget.

6. Suggest that the fee include representation in a tax audit. Some will say okay while others will want to sell you audit insurance. At least get a rough estimate of an audit cost.

7. When choosing between a CPA and a non-certified accountant, you need to know your state's requirements as well as your own needs. If you need certified statements, about half the states require that they be performed by a CPA. If you don't need certified statements—if you have no investors, for example, or your bank doesn't require or ask for them—then a CPA isn't required. In general, CPAs are more knowledgeable as they have more education, but there are plenty of good accountants and enrolled agents as well. Beyond these considerations, choose the individual you feel the most comfortable with.

In the same article in *Independent Business Magazine* (by the way, this is a remarkable magazine chock-full of great tips and ideas for businesses such as ours—subscription info in Appendix A), Howard Scott delineates some pitfalls to avoid in dealing with an accountant:

1. **Paying for excess information.** Information is worthless if you don't use it. If you get regular reports but don't use them to change your business practice—or worse, don't even read them—you don't need the reports. (Or the billing for the time to produce them!)
2. **Making your accountant the scapegoat.** Accountants are advisors, not tricksters. They are not to blame for the normal problems of running a business.
3. **Doing the last minute scramble.** When your accountant steps into your salon, you are on the clock. Have everything—all materials—well organized. Looking for documents and information is an expensive time-waster.
4. **Supplying incomplete information.** Don't withhold or provide inaccurate information. Without a complete and accurate (read true) picture of your business, your accountant may unwittingly tender bad advice.
5. **Ignoring effects on your taxes.** Taxes are a significant aspect of most of your business decisions. Taking into account tax ramifications of a decision can save you a bunch.
6. **Going with the low bidder.** Value is as value gets. What your accountant charges is secondary to what he or she provides. Good accountants are cheap whatever their price. Remember that in today's complex business world, virtually every business decision has an accounting angle, and the expertise necessary to make the right move usually entails an accounting professional.

SETTING UP AN INVENTORY CONTROL SYSTEM

Now you are ready to begin to set up your inventory control system. There are several good systems available, and you may have your own system that works just fine for you. The system described here is only one model and perhaps not the best one for your situation. Your accountant can advise you on what is best for you.

Also, there are many good computer inventory programs, some even as sophisticated as to allow bar coding. Come to think of it, that is not as sophisticated an idea as it was just a few short years ago—some are predicting bar codes everywhere in the very near future. Hospitals are even placing bar codes on donor organs!

Regardless of the inventory system, you will need a way to identify and track items. A standard way is a numbering system, usually a one to five character mnemonic, that represents each item in your inventory. In the model here, we suggest a three-digit system, beginning with the number one hundred. Setting up such a system will make the transition to a computer software program later on much easier, as many of them are based on such numbering systems. Here is how it works, using conditioners as an example:

8 oz. Bold Strokes Moist. Cond.	Inventory Code: 100
16 oz. Bold Strokes Moist. Cond.	101
8 oz. Bold Strokes Reconditioner	102
16 oz. Bold Strokes Reconditioner	103
8 oz. Bold Strokes Cond. for Dry Hair	104
16 oz. Bold Strokes Cond. for Dry Hair	105

You get the idea. Any numbering system you care to use is fine so long as it fits your needs and is logical. When you have all your products numbered, then you need to establish minimum and maximum stock levels, the minimum level representing the number of stock at which you will reorder. A computer system will automatically tally your inventory each time an item is sold, but you can do the same thing manually. It just takes longer! At systematic periods, such as weekly, a physical inventory should be taken of all retail and usage stock, and then a purchase order can be made from those items that have reached your established minimum levels. You can also quickly tell if you are being affected by pilferage and theft and take steps to correct the problem.

Other information in your system should be the distributor, the wholesale unit price, and the retail price.

A count sheet for physically counting inventory should include such information as the inventory code and description, the vendor, minimum/maximum inventory levels, the on-hand count, and the inventory class. An inventory class is a group of items of the same type, such as shampoos. (Figure 6.2)

Some areas that can be computed from inventory figures are total salon sales of a particular product, total sales in a single class, total

FIGURE 6.2
And you think *you* have inventory problems!

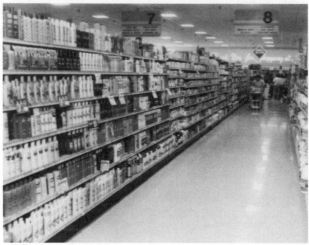

product sales, vendor purchases in a single class, or total vendor purchases. Individual totals can easily be obtained as well. Usage figures will tell you salon total use of a product, of a class of products, overall usage total, and individual totals. When a stylist uses a product at the backbar or at the sink, he or she should check out that item so that you can track it. This is an excellent system to determine waste and overusage of products by stylists.

Comparing sales and usage figures for different periods will give you a clear picture of who is improving in sales and who is declining. Goals may be set realistically, once you know the history and pattern of sales and usage figures, both for the salon and for individual stylists.

Establish a standard period in which to track your products. When you see items are not moving, you can then make some decisions. An item that has been on the shelf for a lengthy period may have to be returned to the vendor for a refund, enabling you to use that sum to purchase another product that moves faster. You may decide to make that item a sale item. You may choose to place it in another location on the shelf to see if that spurs sales. You may feel the best thing to do is to offer your staff additional motive to sell the item, an increased commission or some sort of prize for selling the most. The main thing is, you should be able to see, by proper tracking, that some sort of action is called for, rather than simply allowing the item to remain and collect dust on the shelf.

Track retail sales by stylist as well. Such information should help you see where sales are weak, by individual. If you see Nancy is selling tons of Brand X shampoo, but no conditioners by Brand C, she may simply need some product education so that she sees the benefits and values of the product herself. Conversely, discovering that Nancy is selling prodigious amounts of a particular product or product line may be valuable information in that she may be able to pass on to the rest of the staff tips on how to sell that product. It may be that she is just so enthusiastic about the product herself that it is easy for her to sell it, and you can tap into that zeal by having her give a sales talk on the product's virtues to the rest of your personnel. Enthusiasm for a product has a way of transferring itself to those who come into contact with it.

If you are not computerized, standard inventory sheets are generally available from most manufacturers and distributors. Most distributors will also be happy to conduct regular inventories of their own products for you, keeping you stocked at the levels you establish. A word of caution here; most salespersons are honest and care about your business, but there are those that will want to overstock you—don't allow that to happen. And most distributors should be willing to allow you to return merchandise that isn't moving well. They may require a certain period before they will take back products or have other requirements, such as taking it back for a lesser figure than what you paid initially, and it is not fair to expect them to credit you with a refund at the regular price when you bought it at a sale price (nor will they allow it!). Find out each of your vendor's policies about taking back merchandise before you make your first purchase. If they adopt a hard-line position, you may look for another vendor or another line, and chances are good that you can negotiate from such a stance as well. Generally, most distributors have some sort of take-back policy.

Proper inventory control is something that should not be left to chance. You should not employ the system of ordering in which you only pick up the phone to the supplier when Janie mentions you are down to one bottle of BubbleTickle shampoo! This is suicide. Worse, this is dumb.

Get a handle on what you have in the salon, what is selling, who is selling it, and what is just sitting there, ticking away profits.

REVIEW

Keeping track of inventory may not seem exciting, but keeping an accurate account of your products is very important to the smooth operation of your salon. Too much of a product can eat at your profits; too little can result in lost sales. Three factors determine the profitability of your retail sales: gross sales, gross profit margins, and overhead expenses.

Choosing the right accountant will have both short-term and long-term benefits for your salon. Your accountant can advise you about which inventory control system will be best for you to use.

PRICING STRATEGY

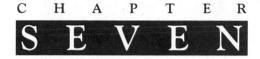

C H A P T E R
SEVEN

How you price your services and retail items could very well prove to be the single most important business decision you make.

That is a strong statement. That is also a very true statement. How you price services and goods will determine not only your profitability, but also the overall attitude of you and your staff. As we are in a people business, attitude is crucial.

One of the unique things about our business is the way individual salons and shops are created. A very typical scenario is this: Stylist goes to school, graduates, finds job with good salon, works hard for five years, establishes a full book, begins to resent portion of commissions paid to employer, opens own salon. Sound like a story you've heard before, perhaps your own story? There's nothing inherently wrong with this; indeed, this is typically the "American way." The flaw with this is in the way we in the hairstyling field traditionally approach opening a salon. Whereas many other businesses are initiated by those with specialized training in general business principles and strategies, even with college degrees or at least with a basic business background obtained by completing rudimentary courses, stylists most of the time take a reverse tack. We open our business with an artistic knowledge and talent, but possess little or no business savvy, so we end up running our salons by the seat of our pants, learning as we go— if we survive long enough to take advantage of often very painful and costly lessons in the world of business.

As a matter of fact, that is the whole purpose of this book—to pass on some of those business tenets that are absolutely essential to success and even survival.

We probably all know of at least one salon owner who enjoyed a tremendous business as far as bookings were concerned. He or she was solidly booked for weeks or even months in advance, but ended up closing the doors or even declaring bankruptcy. How is that possible, we ask ourselves? By not knowing or adhering to the laws of business, by not having sufficient knowledge of all the facets of running a successful business, and by not being aware of or following proven business practices.

And one of the most important elements of establishing a business that will turn a profit, if not the single most important element, is proper pricing.

Here is a situation that is all too common. An ambitious stylist, blessed with talent and a host of loyal clients who will follow the stylist to China if need be, decides it is time to venture off and open the doors to a new salon. The stylist obtains the necessary financing, finds the location, does the remodeling, purchases the equipment, does all the things necessary to open a business, and then sets down to determine the pricing schedule.

At this point, fear sets in. The stylist is acutely aware of the investment involved—the money loaned by the lending institution, friends, family, savings— and all of a sudden becomes aware that failure is a possibility. A phobia, known in gambling circles as "betting the rent money," develops. When you sit down to a poker game, the best way to ensure losing your shirt is to "bet the rent money"; that is, bet money you can't afford to lose. This kind of attitude leads to defeatest moves such as hedging bets, betting too conservatively, betting too aggressively, or, in other words, betting unrealistically. The outcome is foreordained—in poker, at least, that person will end up losing the farm. The same, unfortunately, can be true in the salon business.

Opening a business is a gamble, make no mistake about that. Granted, it is a calculated gamble, one in which one weighs the pros and cons and determines that the positives outweigh the negatives and therefore the business has a reasonable chance to succeed, but all of the best planning in the world still leaves the entrepreneur with a gamble. If there weren't any risks, there wouldn't be any rewards, not substantial rewards anyway.

It is at this point that our fictional stylist makes a common, disastrous mistake. He hedges the bet. Where the stylist had been working, he charged $20 for a basic service, a haircut and style. Now, the stylist becomes unsure, wondering if he will lose substantial numbers of clients, and makes an unwise decision. He decides to open the salon with reduced prices. The stylist has just looked into the mirror and given himself the kiss of death. (If this sounds melodramatic, good.)

The salon opens with a haircut price of $10. The stylist is now playing poker and "betting the rent money," i.e., betting scared. The reasoning has become flawed—"I will charge $10 to be sure I have enough business to cover expenses. Then, when I am busy, and booked ahead, I will raise prices."

The reasoning is not only specious; it is completely short circuited. The stylist has not continued the reasoning applied to its logical end. Let us say that a full booking is achieved with the $10 haircut and style. How does the stylist propose to get the price back up to $20? In one fell swoop wherein the price is doubled? Not likely—not unless the stylist wishes to lose 100 percent of the existing clientele. By raising $2 every six weeks? How many of those "bumps" do you think the average client will stand for? What is the average client going to think when on every revisit to the salon, the charge for a haircut is raised by $2? The client might stick around for two such raises, but will be long gone before the fifth such raise—the one that gets the price to where it should have been originally.

Whatever price you open with is going to be the basic price you will have to live with, except for reasonable periodic raises due to increased supply and demand, inflation, and other traditional and sound reasons for price raises.

And what kind of attitude will our stylist have when charging half of what he feels he is worth, when he first opens? In the first week or even month after opening, in the first flush of owning a business, the stylist won't mind very much. Too shortly, though, this euphoria will wear off, and the stylist will begin to resent the fact that he is charging less than what the work is worth. His attitude will go south, and when attitude sours so does work—prices won't even have to be raised to drive clients away; attitude and quality of work will do that.

Don't make this mistake!

HOW TO SET PRICES

The first consideration in setting prices for your new salon should be to determine what you honestly feel your work to be worth. In many, if not most, instances a price raise is in order. It is hard to imagine a case in which a lower price than what you have been charging is desirable, unless you are planning an entirely different type of salon and an entirely different quality of work.

Pricing services too low is one of the most common mistakes made in pricing. It leads to demoralization, and at some point grim reality is sure to set in. Then the stylist who has offered services for too low a price begins to realize there is no way to get the prices up to where they should be without losing most of the clientele. If an error in pricing strategy is to be made, it is almost invariably better to err high than low.

Pricing services and goods is one area in which you should be full partners with your accountant. Even if you are not about to make the mistake of lowering the price you already charge, on the occasion of opening your own salon, the present price you charge may be too low to achieve a reasonable and fair profit. Only by crunching the numbers can you determine what should be charged, and unless you are a whiz at this, consult your accountant.

Your business plan will be the basis for determining prices when opening a new salon. You will have two sorts of expenses, variable and fixed, which will be primary determining factors in pricing strategy. To begin with, you should calculate what your basic pricing unit is. In most instances, this unit will be your most commonly performed service, usually a haircut or a haircut and style. Assuming this to be the case, you would refer to a haircut as a unit and its cost as the unit price. You then need to determine, as closely as you can, how many units per month you expect to perform and multiply that by unit price. You would do the same for all your other basic units—permanent waves, color services, manicures, all the services offered—and determine what your expected monthly income will be. This is an estimate, but it should be figured as closely as possible. This is not the place for pie-in-the-sky figures (what you hope will happen), but realistic, honest appraisals. Underestimate, if anything. The figure you and your accountant come up with must match or exceed your breakeven figure, unless you have predetermined a period of time in which you expect to operate at a loss and have provided for such in your planning. If you determine it will cost you $2,000 per month in operating costs, and you estimate you will only bring in $1,500 in revenue, it doesn't take a rocket scientist to figure out where the business is headed. If, in your estimation, this will be the case, it is time to make some serious adjustments in your business plan, or else you are probably headed for trouble. You would need to eliminate or drastically reduce basic expenses, in this instance, or come up with a way to generate additional income.

The sample chart will give you an idea of how to estimate and determine profitability:

Fixed Expenses Per Month
(Figures Are Rounded)

Rent	$ 850.00
Utilities	600.00
Wages (One-person salon)	2,000.00
Debt Service (See Amortization Sched.)	1,384.76
Accounting, legal, phone, office supplies	275.00
Taxes, SS, Workers' Compensation	450.00
Insurances	75.00
Refuse Pickup	50.00
Total Fixed Expenses	$5,684.76

Variable Expenses Per Month

Advertising	$ 450.00
Use Supplies	500.00
Retail Supplies (Avg. 50% markup)	650.00
Total Variable Expenses	$1,600.00
*Total Expenses	$8,134.76

*Total Expenses—This figure represents the breakeven point.

SALES PROJECTIONS

Breakeven Sales: This figure is the total of my anticipated business operating expenditures, which is $8,134.76 per month. I estimate services to account for 85% of required revenues, initially, which would be $6,914.55. As my basic service unit (haircut and style) is priced at $30, I need to generate 230 unit sales monthly, providing 85% of necessary revenues. Approximately $1,200 in additional income is to be realized from retail sales, which provides the remaining 15% of revenues.

This is just a basic view of how you achieve your breakeven point and tells you what you have to achieve in sales to at least make expenses. Please don't use the categories and/or figures shown here in computing your own. Your sales projection figures should include all expected sales such as permanent waves, color, highlightings, facials—any and all services to be offered. Expenses should include all costs as well, which should be much more detailed than the example given here. This is exhibited only to give you a general outline of how to proceed in compiling your own figures. An accountant is invaluable and will probably have a more exact way of computing not only what your breakeven point will be, but what you should be charging for each service.

PRICING RETAIL PRODUCTS

Charges for retail items are sometimes taken for granted, inasmuch as most distributors and product companies have suggested retail prices that most salons adhere to. Although these suggested prices are handy in assigning a price to a particular item, such as an eight-ounce bottle of shampoo, don't take for granted that you will realize a profit at that price. Again, your accountant can help you determine what the proper pricing should be. Most companies suggest a markup of 40–50 percent. (This can be confusing, as some companies say that when you buy an item from them for $1 and sell it for $2, this is a 50 percent markup; others call this a 100 percent markup.) This is only a matter of mathematical semantics—what is important is that the markup percentage used be profitable to you. How can it be unprofitable to buy something for $1 and sell it for $2? Sounds impossible, doesn't it? Well, sorry to say, it's not. It's very possible to have such a markup on items and lose money.

There are more expenses involved in the retail sale of a bottle of shampoo than the cost of the shampoo itself. This is an area, again, where your accountant can definitely be extremely useful.

Besides the actual cost of the bottle of shampoo, there are some other very real costs as well. Do you pay a sales commission to your stylists when they sell products? If so, that must be figured as part of the expense of that unit. How long it sits on the shelf before it is taken by a customer is part of the cost in several ways. For one thing, the bottle of shampoo that sits unsold on the shelf for any length of time has an interest loss for that period. If you paid $4 for a bottle of shampoo expecting to sell it for $8, and it didn't sell for six months, you have to add the amount of interest that $4 would have earned in a standard investment, such as a savings account or other such instrument. That is part of the cost of the item to you. By simply depositing that money in the bank, you would have earned that much in a conservative investment, more in another investment instrument. This is part of the cost of doing business, especially retail business.

There is another hidden cost. The shampoo took up some room on the shelf, and therefore room in the salon space on which you are paying rent and overhead. Even if you own the building, there is a depreciation factor at work—somewhere, no matter what the situation, it costs you very real dollars for your retail space, and items that don't move in a reasonable period of time cost you a lot. You need to figure your shelf storage and display costs to arrive at the proper pricing.

Yet another cost is maintenance. Does someone dust and/or clean your shelves and retail items on a regular basis? If so, a wage cost is involved, as well as a portion of all the other employee costs. Could their time have been spent more profitably on another activity?

You can start to see that what looks to be a simple chore— pricing a bottle of shampoo—becomes much more complex than it appears, especially if you wish the item for sale to turn a profit. Don't despair. Your accountant can be of tremendous help. He or she is very aware of and familiar with all the costs we've covered and others. In retail sales, very standard and accepted costs are involved in the pricing strategy, and it is a rare bean-counter who cannot help you here.

A closely watched inventory is tremendously necessary to assure profitability. In chapter 6 we covered this subject in more detail. Suffice to say, retail pricing is not a cut and dried procedure where you blindly follow the manufacturer's or distributor's recommendation or suggested prices.

Let us say that you invested $4 in a bottle of Salon Ecstasy shampoo from your friendly dealer on 1/1/90, and finally sold it to Mr. Z on 1/1/91 for $8, the suggested retail price. (Figure 7.1) You made $4, right? If you've read this far, you know that's wrong. You probably knew that was wrong long before you read this, but perhaps didn't know how much you actually made. If you knew what your retail costs were, you could very quickly add it up. Let's see how that works. While we're at it, let's throw another figure into the equation—let's say you noticed that bottle had been hanging around for ten months and wasn't selling, so you placed it on sale at 10 percent off. Your net profit or loss on the bottle of shampoo would look something like this:

Initial Cost of Product	$ 4.00
Loss of interest on money invested (8%)	.32
Stylist's sales commission (15%)	.60
Rent & Overhead (item took 1/5,000th of space)	.27
Maintenance (Receptionist unwrapped it, stocked it on the shelf, put a price tag on it, replaced it once when it came off, cleaned the item once a week for 52 weeks, figured up the new sale price, rang up the sale, and placed it in the retail bag. Total time she spent—23 minutes. Receptionist is paid $6.00 per hour.)	2.30
Retail bag	.10
Total Cost of Item	$ 7.59
Sold for: $8.00 minus 10% (sale price) =	7.20
Therefore, the item sold for a *loss* of	$ .39

FIGURE 7.1
Are you sure you sold that item at a profit?

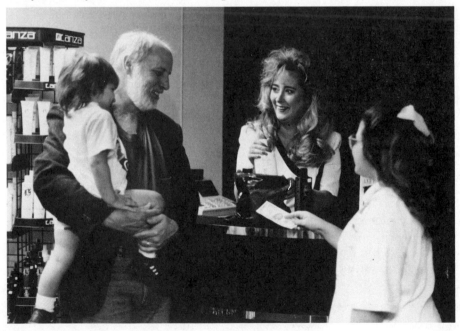

Yes, that's right. You lost $.39 the day the item was sold. The only one who made anything on the sale (other than the manufacturer and the distributor) was the stylist who sold it. Hopefully, that was you and not one of your hired guns! Does this help make it clearer how important proper pricing is? It should!

The first time these costs were brought to my own attention, I invented a new word that fully described how I felt. The word was "dismazed" and is a combination of the words *dismayed* and *amazed*. I think it an entirely appropriate new addition to any stylist's vocabulary, and it is surprising how many times in this business that I have been dismazed to the hilt! Haven't you?

Realizing all the hidden costs of retailing should tell the salon owner something else—to keep a close eye on what is moving reasonably quickly and what is not and to eliminate those items that just sit and collect dust on the shelves (or have the dust removed many times by a paid employee).

Also, it seems important and prudent that the salon owner and all of his or her distributors work together in having an agreement that items not moving be allowed to be returned or exchanged for full value. A distributor that refuses to take back products may be of questionable value to your business, and it may be worthwhile to locate another, more flexible dealer for the products you require. If another one cannot be located, and the original dealer remains intractable, you might call the manufacturer of the product and let them know your situation. Most reputable distributors and dealers have a take-back policy, knowing it is not to the benefit of either party to have you stuck with products that are going to take forever to move. If you happen to have a dealer who won't work with you on this, sometimes the manufacturer can suggest a remedy or put the necessary pressure on the distributor to deal with you in a more businesslike fashion.

PRICING SERVICES

Just as we've seen in the pricing of retail items, the pricing of services has many components to consider. The bottom line is the bottom line. The paramount reason for any business to be in existence is to create a profit for the owners. If along the way jobs are created for others, then that is good, but that is not the reason business exists. If the owner does not keep that goal solidly before him or her, and the business ceases to turn a reasonable profit, then there simply won't be any jobs—unless, of course, the owner has an unlimited supply of dollar bills, which is not often the case.

When many of us began in the styling business years ago, it wasn't uncommon for commissions paid to stylists to average 70 percent and, in some cases, even higher. Today, in commission payment schemes, percentages paid to the stylist are down to 50, 40, and in some instances, even as low as 35 percent. Salons that refused to adjust to the financial realities of today's conditions found their doors being closed.

Over and over, I keep bringing up the profession of accounting, but that is only because your accountant is probably the most important person in your business. Because the world of commerce today is so complex, the services of such a professional are not a luxury of the bigger salons; they are an absolute necessity for survival. We can no longer go by the established traditional methods of payment to employees and pricing of services and goods and expect to compete in a business sense with other salons more attuned to the realities of the marketplace. The only thing constant in life (and in business) is change, and the salon of today must accommodate those changes or join the failed salons of yesteryear.

Work hand-in-hand with your accountant to determine just exactly what your price structure should be to provide a profit; attract new business; keep yourself and stylists you hire motivated, happy, and feeling they are paid what their work is worth; and assure you are well on your way to having a business that will remain healthy. And wealthy!

SOME FOOD FOR THOUGHT

There is another element of the pricing equation I failed to mention—competitors' prices. There are times and situations when what your competitors charge is very important. It hasn't been mentioned until now because many times what the salon down the street charges seems to be the *only* determinant involved in affixing prices, and it is a very poor factor in pricing decisions. Chances are better than good that your competitor hasn't thought out his or her own pricing strategy very well, and you could be following the lead of someone who is perilously close to financial disaster.

And too, our business is not like many other businesses, such as the tool and die business, the fast food business, or the supermarket business. We have a wide diversity of talents, abilities, images, and, therefore, prices.

Rather than let what others charge take an elevated position in your priorities in establishing prices, it may be better to adhere to the philosophy of Indiana University men's basketball coach, Bobby Knight. His teams don't play "other teams"; they "play against themselves"— against the high standards they have set for their own performance. If they do that, Knight says, they will usually win.

The same philosophy can work for hairstylists. If you always work to the best of your ability, then charge the price you think fair for that work—*not* the price your competitor charges. Just be honest and fair with your appraisal of yourself. It is an excellent bet that if you truly feel your haircut is worth $30, clients will agree. If you feel your work is worth $30 and you charge only $20, how do you think you will begin to feel about that? Most people who are paid less than what they perceive themselves and their work to be worth end up lowering the quality of that work to where it matches the payment given. It's funny how perceptions influence reality. My wife and business partner, Mary, has a saying that best describes many underachievers, not only in our business, but in life in general. Her way of putting it is that the person in question "keeps bumping his head on his own ceiling."

Of course take into account what competitors are charging in determining your own pricing schedule—but not to the detriment of your own business. And be sure the person whose prices you take into consideration is, indeed, a competitor and not just someone who has a salon in the near geographical proximity. Even if they are located next door, they may very well not be "competitors" at all, any more than McDonald's is a competitor with the dining room at the Ritz-Carlton. They are competitors only in the sense that they both serve edible substances, but the market they are after is vastly different. This is not meant to be a pejorative comparison of either McDonald's or the Ritz-Carlton's dining room—both are hugely successful in attracting the market they have attempted to serve, and one is not "better" than the other, any more than a higher-priced salon is "better" than a budget salon.

If you are using other salons' prices to determine your own, compare only salons of quality equal to your own (equate apples to apples, not apples to oranges). When you have identified those, go even further, and use your best educated judgment as to whether those prices will lead to profitability.

Another factor at work in pricing is psychological. Whether it is true or not, many people equate quality with price. If it costs more, it is better. We all know that not to be a 100 percent true statement, but don't you believe it yourself, most of the time? How many times have you heard, "You get what you pay for"? (How many times have you said it yourself?)

Several years ago, I was forced by circumstances and a family situation to make several moves in a year's time, which resulted in my working in three different salons in two different states. In each salon I charged a different haircut price—in the first my haircuts cost $40, in the second $22, and in the third $30. Quite a range in prices, and each salon was successful. At all three salons I performed my work at the same level of quality, which was simply to the best of my knowledge and ability. The only variable was the price. There is a lot of difference between charging $22 and $40 for the same service; the difference was not in the haircut, but in the perception of the client receiving the service. That is the psychological factor at work in pricing. The prices are meaningless—to some stylists those would have seemed high, to others low—but in each salon the clientele considered the prices fair.

Don't make the mistake of overlooking the psychological factor in deciding on what to charge. As in any other business, you charge what the market will bear. If the marketplace doesn't feel you're worth what you charge, you'll find this out readily. It is your job as a business owner to convince enough members of the buying public that the services offered by you or your salon are worth the price affixed to them.

A psychological factor is at work in any business with an artistic element to it—you can even call it the "snob effect," and it works both ways. Some clients love to drop the name (and prices) of their salon. Others do the same for more budget-minded enterprises for almost the same reasons—to show that they are superior in not being foolish enough to pay exorbitant fees. It can work both ways for different markets. As fair-minded individuals, we may not like these very human qualities, but as business owners, we should be aware that they exist and take advantage of them.

As small business owners, we don't have the resources giant conglomerates have, but if we keep our eyes and ears open, we can steal their very expensive ideas and strategies.

For instance, reverse snob appeal is being used with great effectiveness in a recent spate of television commercials selling home permanent kits. The general thrust of the ads is that people who spend a comparatively smaller amount for their home perms are highly intelligent in doing so. The ad elevates reverse snobbery to new heights and is, I assume, highly effective. Locally, a leading upscale salon has taken a different tack, showing a woman with a hair disaster she purportedly obtained from using a (nameless) home permanent, and then showing a gorgeous, sophisticated style another woman received from the pricey salon. Again, I assume the ad to be as effective for them as the national ad was for the home perm company, both appealing to different sets of clients, but ostensibly for the same reasons—a form of snobbery, direct or reverse.

Don't discount the psychology of prices in your own stragegy. And don't let other salons have undue influence in the setting of your own prices.

RAISING PRICES

One area of pricing that seems to be sensitive with many stylists and salon owners is price raises. As stylists, we tend to be friends with our clientele, and sometimes this can cause a problem when it comes time to raise prices. We feel such a move may alienate our client/friend, and this attitude may serve to keep us from raising prices when necessary and called for, or may cause us to not raise prices to a level that ensures a profit for the salon.

Unfortunately, there is an element of truth to the supposition that you will lose friends and/or clients if you raise prices. There is little doubt that you lose at least a small percentage.

But you're engaged in a business, and the primary rule of any business is that it must take in more than goes out. The closer the intake figure gets to the outgo figure, the closer a business is to financial ruin. Periodic price raises are necessary and vital to the health of your business. If your "friends" don't understand this, then perhaps their brand of friendship is too costly. You might ask yourself how many of those so called friends would be there to bail you out if you were forced to close your salon doors because you failed to increase your prices when needed.

It's a hard thing for some to accept, but you must divorce

friendship from business. This sort of friendship is not real in the first place, being a one-sided relationship, and not sufficiently respectful of your professionalism and your right to earn a living at that profession.

More than one salon has been forced to close its doors for no other reason than the owner putting off raising prices when it was the correct time to implement such a decision—because of a misguided desire to salve supposed client displeasure, which may have never materialized at all.

STAFF PRICING

Another area you should look at very carefully when determining your fee schedule is what stylists in your employ will be charging. Common practice in the majority of salons is for each stylist in the same salon to charge basically the same price, the price list reflecting salon prices and not individual stylist's prices. Chances are this has been the situation at the shop(s) or salon(s) at which you have worked, as the majority of salons price their services this way.

However, if you look closely, this system has several flaws. First, it would be nice if all stylists were equal in ability, but the fact is that we are not. Even if we were, the buying public would perceive differences simply because of personality. This may not seem fair, but it is a fact of life. The reality is that we all have differing degrees of ability, experience, and talent. To insist that all the stylists in a salon charge the same price is to pretend that these differences don't exist.

In truth, many salons that post the same service fees for all their stylists are being unfair to their stylists and clientele alike. It puts the stylist in the uncomfortable position of having to perform at a level he or she is not yet capable of. This many times causes the stylist to fib to the client about his or her experience level—not a situation conducive to establishing professional trust, especially when it is obvious the stylist has not yet attained the plateau claimed.

If the stylist in this situation opts for truth, building a clientele will be a long, slow process. This, in effect, penalizes truth-telling. Doesn't this sound like a familiar scenario in many salons?

One of the myths that abound within our industry says it takes a year or two years to build a clientele. As with many old wives' tales, there is a kernel of truth involved. It takes that long to build a clientele if the salon approach to pricing is as described above (and, it takes that long to build a clientele if the stylist *believes* it will take that long—recall our own warning that many create their own ceilings to bump their heads on). If you, as a salon owner, hire an inexperienced stylist or one with a decidedly lower level of ability than others in the salon, and insist he or she charge the same price as the others, you are probably dooming that person to a long period of inactivity. You may refuse to acknowledge differences in ability levels, but you can bet the client will notice.

This gets us to the other side of the chair—the side the client sits on. Is it fair to expect clients to pay the same price to each stylist within the salon, if there are significant differences in ability? Of course not. You, as the owner, may claim that all your stylists are of equal ability, but the people coming in your doors will react differently. If the salon price is $20 for a haircut and style regardless of who performs the service, who do you think will end up with the most clients? That's easy—the stylist(s) who appear to offer to the buyer the best value for the money.

It's just not fair to expect clients to pay the same fee for unequal value. It's just not fair to expect a stylist to try and perform at a level not yet obtained.

There are several ways out of this dilemma. Many successful salons use a level system, in which stylists are assigned a level, based on salon criteria that take into account several factors, and each level within the salon has corresponding prices. Stylists in each level have a clear, defined means of achieving the next highest level.

In our own salon, we have created a system of three levels, which we designate co-designer, designer, and senior designer. Each level has a set of requirements that must be met before advancing to the next level, and each has a different service fee schedule. When a stylist meets the requirements for the next level and is promoted, he or she gains not only a deserved raise, due to the increase in prices, but also a sense of accomplishment that goes with achieving something difficult. Our promotions are not given; they are hard earned and well deserved.

We make certain that our clients are aware of our level system and also how difficult it is for the stylist to advance, explaining exactly what is involved in this procedure. Then, when stylists are promoted, most of their clients go with them, gladly paying the price increase—most feel a proprietary interest in "their" stylists, like they have helped them along in their advancement (which they have!). This system works well for both stylist and client, and is fair to both sides of the chair.

A level system does several other things. It improves staff morale tremendously. It tells stylists that they are involved in a career, not just a job, and there are steps to take that will broaden their professional knowledge and abilities, thereby increasing their value to both themselves and the salon. It gives stylists a tremendous sense of pride and accomplishment. Advancing to the next level is not an automatic thing that will occur with enough seniority. We "big-dealize" each promotion by running ads in the local newspaper, putting up banners in the salon, and sending the newly promoted stylist flowers and a cake. Why? Because it *is* a big deal—the stylist has earned the promotion!

Studies find that most job dissatisfaction stems not from employees being underpaid, but from a sense of not being appreciated or valued. I have given many pay raises to employees over the years and cannot recall a single instance in which the employee was so grateful he or she cried. I have had many, many experiences similar to the one I shared with thirty-four-year-old Grace (fictitious name) who, upon being promoted, came to me with tears in her eyes and said it was the first time in her life she had had to work so hard and also the first time she had felt appreciated for what she had done.

Creating a level system does something else for your staff. It affords them the opportunity to remove the ceiling from their income, allowing them to make whatever the market will bear. Each price level in our salon is always designated as a minimum price, which may be higher depending on factors such as length of hair and extra time necessary for the service. Minimum prices are posted for senior designers, but each stylist who has attained our highest level charges different prices, depending on the demand for that person's services.

This is the way it works: When a senior designer has consistently been booked three months ahead for at least three months, that stylist's prices are raised 10 percent. Then, when the stylist again meets that criterion, prices are raised once more. That stylist can charge whatever the market will bear and has, in effect, removed the ceiling from his or her income.

Which leads us neatly to the final subject of this chapter.

When Is a Price Raise Justified?

There are only two conditions when prices should (and must) be raised. One: When it is necessary to provide a profit. Two: When the market will bear it.

In the first instance, as a business person, you must maintain a pricing strategy that will return more money back to the salon than what you pay out. If the cost of business goes up, so must the prices, and it is inevitable, given our economic system, that costs will go up. Included in business costs is inflation, which is only the cost of money appreciating. A price raise because of increases in business costs is easy—if it cost you 10 percent more to operate your salon this year than it did the year before, then you need to raise your prices at least 10 percent to stay even. If your profit margin wasn't where you wanted it, perhaps you need an even higher raise.

This is pretty cut and dry. Costs go up, prices go up. Simple. What is not so simple is deciding when and how much to raise prices in the second condition, because of supply and demand.

One way of determining how high you can safely raise service prices is the method we use in our own salon and described earlier, in which senior designers' prices are raised each time they book ahead consistently for a predetermined period of time (in our case, three months). Something like this may work well for you, or you may prefer to come up with your own system. Be sure to keep in mind that one or two raises a year will ordinarily not scare away clientele, provided that clientele does not view those raises as excessive, but more frequent price changes than that tend to increasingly offend more people.

One thing is sure, however. No matter what percentage of clientele is lost due to an increase, the salon is ahead of the game if the gross intake remains the same or increases. For instance, if you raise prices 10 percent, and lose 5 percent of your business by doing so, then you have made a net gain of 5 percent. It is always a goal of business to do less work for more money—this is the primary goal of both labor and management and is not a negative thing. Doing less work for more reward is one of the prime means by which societies and civilizations advance.

The service part of our business is dependent upon the factor of time, which is finite. There are only so many hours in the day, week, month, year, and only so many working hours available to us. Therefore, we must find ways to maximize production within the time factor. Charging what the market will bear is the best way to achieve this.

Those who have been hesitant about raising prices in the past will discover something curious when they begin to get their fees up to where they should be. Their clientele will begin to look at them with respect. If you give your work away, so to speak, you usually also give away the respect for your work.

Another curious fact. I've worked in many different types of salons, with all kinds of prices, and although my own work remained the same, the higher-priced salon for some reason always seemed to attract the less-demanding client. Those who have always worked in lower-priced and budget salons sometimes have the mistaken notion that if they were to charge a higher price the client would become more picky, but in my own experience the opposite is true. The lower the price, the more the client demanded, and many of those demands were ridiculous. I think the reason for that is the lack of respect given the stylist charging too low a fee. Many clients assume that if their stylist charges a cheaper fee for the service, he or she must not be very good and, therefore, they have to instruct the stylist in every phase of the job. The same client in a higher-priced salon doesn't say a word, but accepts the work done and offers back not criticism and demands, but high praise.

I've asked, in a sort of informal, unscientific poll, many stylists in many different types of salons what kind of clientele their salons attracted, and it is my honest feeling that the more charged for their services, the less demanding the clientele.

To recap, be certain that the prices charged for both retail items and services are fair to both parties, and enough to ensure a profit. In determining prices, be certain to include all factors, not just the wholesale cost of the product. In services, as well, be certain to include all costs and factors in your determinations. Remember, you cannot compare what you earn per hour to most other industries, trades, or professions, especially to those individuals who earn a salary, as they earn far more than just their hourly wage—they also are normally given a benefits package. Health insurances, dental and eyeglass insurances, pension plans, profit-sharing programs, paid holidays and vacations, paid sick days, life insurance programs, pregnancy leaves— the list of benefits many other workers receive seems to go on and on. The stylist normally has none of these benefits others seem to take for granted. We have to purchase our own benefits, usually at a higher cost. This, too, must be calculated in order to arrive at equitable prices for our services.

In the seventies, I happened to be in a city where one of the major manufacturing factories was leaving town, relocating for cheaper labor.

The local newspaper published the average salary and benefits package for the employees of that concern, including all wage hour earners, from the lowest to the highest paid. Average yearly salaries were roughly $26,000, and average yearly benefits packages were worth roughly $18,000! That figure was mind-boggling to me, as my total benefits at the time amounted to a health insurance policy with a ridiculously high deductible that I paid for out of my own pocket. A sweeper in a factory was getting $18,000 a year in benefits—and probably grousing about paying too much for his or her haircut!

Be sure to include the cost of your own benefits package in your price schedule. If you don't, you won't get one!

And educate your clients. You don't have to cry the blues to them, and you shouldn't, but most people are unaware of how small business works. All many of them see are what they presume you are making per hour (based on the service you perform on them divided into a forty-hour week and multiplied). Here is exactly what a client will do. You cut his or her hair in half an hour and charge $30; he or she will mentally calculate that you therefore make $60 an hour, which, times forty hours, equals $2,400 per week. The client doesn't realize you may not be 100 percent booked, all services may not be priced according to this schedule, and you had six no-shows this week alone, four of them for three-hour highlights! No, all the client will "know" is that you make a heck of a lot more per hour than he or she does. Explaining a little about how business actually works, if done in the right way, can go a long way toward client acceptance of prices.

The other thing about the factory's benefits package was that I couldn't have purchased the same package for the same price. They had the group buying power of five thousand employees. I would have had to purchase it as an individual, which means the same package would have cost me at least half again what it had the factory.

The purpose of all this is not to vent sour grapes, but to be sure you realize all that should be included in your pricing formula. Again, a good accountant is invaluable in calculating your prices, and a much better source than merely following the lead of a neighboring salon that very probably is grossly underpriced.

And underpricing your products and services is simply the kiss of death in any business venture. Don't doom your salon before it even has a chance to succeed.

REVIEW

How you price your services and retail items may be the single most important business decision you make. The business plan will be the basis for determining prices in a new salon. An accountant will provide valuable information that will help price each service and item.

Your competitors' prices should be a factor—but not the only factor—in your own pricing structure. Compare only the prices in salons of equal quality to your own, and use your own educated judgment to determine whether those prices will lead to profitability.

BOOKKEEPING

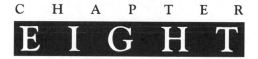

EIGHT

The word *bookkeeping* inevitably draws a groan—the listener visualizes a scene in which hour upon tedious hour is spent, late at night, poring over rows and columns of numbers and figures with complicated designations like post-closing trial balances and contra assets. What the heck—we're artists, not nose-to-the-grindstone bean-counters!

Well, that's certainly one way to look at and approach the bookkeeping function, but another view of this activity might be to see it for what it really is—the method by which we keep score of our business. Pictured in this manner, keeping track of our salon business can become fun and even exciting, especially once we see how we can make the business even more profitable, which is one of the primary products of bookkeeping. And, with computers on the scene, the tedium of yesteryear is largely gone. Erase that outdated mental picture of Charles Dickens' Ebenezer Scrooge and Bob Cratchit poring over dusty books on Christmas Eve, for those days are gone forever!

If you haven't yet been introduced to the science of keeping the books, don't create mental blocks and fears that prevent you from approaching the task in a positive way.

There is an old story accountants like to tell about the bookkeeper for a family-owned business, who had been keeping the business records for thirty years. The employees whispered that Miss Elsie knew every secret in the company and that the firm would have a hard time functioning without her knowledge and expertise. Every day, before beginning the morning's work, Miss Elsie would take a key attached to a cord around her neck and secreted in her bosom, unlock the top drawer on her desk, and look intently inside, allowing no one to see what she was inspecting. She would then relock the drawer and get on with the day's activities. When she finally passed away, the first thing interested workers did was break open the drawer and peek inside. (Figure 8.1) Nothing was found except a small slip of paper on which was written in fading ink:

DEBITS GO ON THE LEFT—CREDITS ON THE RIGHT

Perhaps bookkeeping is not this simple, but then it is not as difficult as you may imagine, either. Basically, bookkeeping is merely a system whereby you keep track of the money that changes hands in the

FIGURE 8.1
Bookkeeping is an important part of salon management.

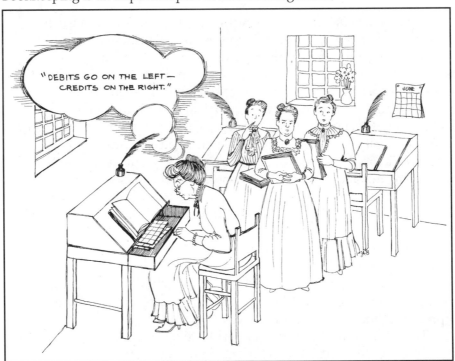

salon—how much came in, how much went out, what you owe, what is owed you, what you own, and how much you are making (or losing). It is a system of recording every transaction. Every monetary transaction requires an entry, and every transaction will eventually be both a credit and a debit. This is referred to as the double-entry method of bookkeeping. Deciding to credit or debit an item is the most common source of confusion to beginning bookkeepers. A good axiom to remember is that any item credited in one place must show as a debit somewhere else.

HELP WITH BOOKKEEPING

I have recommended the services of a professional accountant in much of this book, but this is nowhere as necessary as in your bookkeeping tasks. Even if you perform most of the bookkeeping chores yourself, utilize an accountant to at least set up and monitor your system. Whatever you pay him or her will be money wisely spent. And investigate computers and software systems. Much of the daily routine of maintaining your records can be made immensely easier with the modern, relatively inexpensive software systems now available. Personally, I can recommend QuickBooks by Intuit. *PC Magazine* gives this accounting package its highest marks. It is extremely user-friendly, and you don't have to know or understand double-entry bookkeeping— all you have to know is how to fill out a check. It works just like a checkbook, and even though it is a single-entry system of keeping the books, it will print out double-entry-based reports that are required by banks and accountants. For salons that are computerized, accounting software such as QuickBooks is easy to use, and the planning information it provides is quite sophisticated.

This chapter will introduce you to the basics of bookkeeping and is intended as an overview, not an in-depth study of the subject. For that, you need to consult a professional, such as a bookkeeper, an accountant, your bank, or other financial organization, who can advise you on systems and methods.

A number of good texts are available that delve deeper into the science of bookkeeping. One of the best texts to be found is *Bookkeeping Made Simple* (Louis W. Fields, rev. by Richard R. Gallagher, D.B.A., Doubleday, 1956, 1990), which is quite possibly the finest basic text available and one I highly recommend. Much of the information in this chapter derives from this very easy-to-read and understand book. It explains the double-entry method of bookkeeping.

THE DOUBLE-ENTRY METHOD OF BOOKKEEPING

The principal instrument you will be using is the journal, in which transactions are entered chronologically. That entry is termed making a journal entry. The journal is the daily diary and is the starting place for all bookkeeping. It is the book of original entry. Journal entries are then transferred to other records called accounts, that process called posting, and from those accounts are prepared all kinds of reports that will be valuable to your business. All entries are recorded as either a debit or a credit.

There are several methods of bookkeeping—the one we will present here is the double-entry method, which is the easiest to learn and probably the best for your salon. If your accountant disagrees, listen, as he or she will have close personal knowledge of your salon on which to base the recommendation.

You will need to know two kinds of financial statements. The balance sheet shows what the salon owns (assets), what it owes (liabilities), and what you would have remaining if you paid all you owe out of everything you own (the capital). The operating statement (profit and loss) lists income over a period of time and subtracts expenses to determine a profit or loss.

Assets are what the salon owns and are listed as such whether they are fully paid for or not. For instance, you have a styling chair valued at $800. You paid $400 down and are making payments on the rest. That chair would be listed as an asset, valued at $800, and the remaining balance of $400 would be listed as a liability. A liability is a legal claim against the salon held by someone else.

The basic principle of bookkeeping is that what is owned must be balanced by what is owed. This is called the balance sheet equation, and is expressed thusly:

$$\text{Assets} = \text{Equities}$$

$$\text{Assets} \quad = \quad \underset{\text{(Creditors' Equity)}}{\text{Liabilities}} \quad + \quad \underset{\text{(Owner's Equity)}}{\text{Capital}}$$

TABLE OF DEBITS & CREDITS SHOWING NORMAL ACCOUNT BALANCES

Category of Account	If the transaction increases the account enter a . . .	If the transaction decreases the account enter a . . .	The normal balance is a . . .
Asset	debit	credit	debit
Liability	credit	debit	credit
Capital (Owner's Equity)	credit	debit	credit
Revenue	credit	debit	credit
Expenses	debit	credit	debit

This basic accounting equation is usually abbreviated to $A = L + C$. All it means is that assets must equal equities, which consist of liabilities (creditors' equity) plus capital (owner's equity).

Revenues and expenses must be figured into the formula as well. Revenues are the salon's earnings, from the sale of both services and products. Expenses are what it costs you to do business, and are the expenditures of assets. When expenses are subtracted from revenues, what is left is net income. This cannot be strictly construed as profit, for profit takes several forms. Profit can be gross profit, net profit, or profit before or after taxes. Net income is just what is left after expenses have been paid, and is what we refer to as the bottom line. As a formula, net income appears as follows:

$$R - E = NI$$
$$\text{(revenues)} - \text{(expenses)} = \text{(net income)}$$

The operating statement, or profit and loss statement, is a summary of revenue, expenses, and net income for a period of time, usually either a month, quarter, half-year, or year. A sample operating statement is shown on page 124.

THE ACCOUNTING CYCLE

Bookkeeping has a time frame that is cyclic, and is known as the accounting cycle. This cycle begins with every transaction. Each transaction changes one or more accounts. All accounts must be checked for accuracy (trial balance) as often as needed, at least once each business year and preferably much more often. The closer check you keep on

BOLD STROKES HAIR DESIGN
Operating Statement for the year 1995

REVENUES			
Services revenue		$365,000	
Sales revenue (products)		137,000	
	Total Revenues		$502,000
EXPENSES			
Wages		$286,000	
Rent		20,000	
Insurances		15,000	
Taxes		66,000	
Products		20,000	
Advertising		35,000	
	Total Expenses		$442,000
NET INCOME			$60,000

your business, the better and more accurate forecasts you will be able to make, and the sooner you can spot any potential trouble in the salon business. For the trial balance you will prepare a worksheet in which you summarize the changes in balance sheets and operating statements, making necessary adjustments and entries for changes that are not supported by documentation such as check stubs or sales receipts. Then, you close the books to prepare for the next cycle.

THE JOURNAL

The journal is where all of this starts; as was said before, all transactions are chronologically entered here, as they happen. The journal is also referred to as the book of original entry. You work with records such as dealers' invoices, bank deposit records, and sales slips. Each time you make a recording of a transaction, you are making an entry—in the double-entry system, each transaction is recorded twice, as a credit to one account and a debit to another. To balance the books, the total of all debits must equal the total of all credits. If not, you know an error has been made, an advantage of the double-entry method.

According to *Bookkeeping Made Simple,* you should remember these rules:

- Assets *increase* with debits and *decrease* with credits.
- Liabilities (creditors' equity) *increase* with credits and *decrease* with debits.
- Capital (owner's equity) *increases* with credits and *decreases* with debits.
- Revenues *increase* with credits and *decrease* with debits.
- Expenses *increase* with debits and *decrease* with credits.

This is a handy guide to remember until you are certain of the rules for entering debits and credits in entries. Whenever a transaction is recorded, you must consider:

- What accounts are affected by the entry? (This could be more than one.)
- Are these accounts assets, liabilities, capital, revenues, or expenses?
- Does the transaction increase or decrease them?
- Does this information call for a debit entry or a credit entry?

Here's an example: Suppose you took in $20,000 for the week in service income. You would think this way: "Since I know the event involves cash sales, I know cash is an asset and sales is a revenue. I see that cash (an asset) is increased, and sales (a revenue) is likewise increased. An increase in an asset calls for a debit, while an increase in a revenue calls for a credit." Thus, your journal would balance.

Sometimes a transaction involves more than two accounts. Let's say you bought six new styling chairs for $3,500, paying $1,000 down, signing a promissory note for the balance of $2,500. In this example, two lines are used to record the two credits. The total of these credits should equal the total of the debits. These entries would look like this:

BOLD STROKES HAIR DESIGN
General Journal

19– –	P/R	Debit (Dr.)	Credit (Cr.)
April 1	Styling chairs	$3,500	$1,000
	Note payable to		2,500
	purchase chairs		

Journal entries are entered chronologically; therefore, they are mixed, so now they need to be transferred to a ledger, or a book of accounts in which each type of transaction is recorded—this new record is called an account. For instance, a ledger should have a separate page for cash transactions so you can know the status of cash at all times.

Remember, the process of recording journal entries is called entering. The process of transferring these entries to the appropriate account is termed posting. Since accounts in the ledger take the form of the letter T, they are known as ledger T accounts, similar to journal T accounts in that the left column is the debit (Dr.) side and the right the credit (Cr.) side.

Each journal line has to be posted in the corresponding ledger account. If you sold, say, a wig on November 12 for $85, the cash entry of $85 would be posted as a debit on your cash account ledger page and a credit on your sales revenue account.

There are several common kinds of errors in bookkeeping, and if you have done much bookkeeping at all, you will have probably encountered all of them. A common error is to transpose numbers when entering, recording a ninety-six for a sixty-nine. This kind of mistake is called a transposition error. All such errors are multiples of nine. If you show you are out of balance and the difference between debits and credits is nine or evenly divided by nine, look for a transposition error.

A slide error is one in which you mistakenly move a number over one place, entering 20,000 instead of 2,000 or 200,000. A discrepancy of a large even number should alert you to a slide error.

Other errors are made by failing to post a number or by posting the same number twice. Look at debits and credits to see if there is an entry exactly equal to the discrepancy. If that fails, see if the error divides equally by two, and if it does, look for a duplicate debit or credit posting where there should only be one. A credit may have been posted as a debit or the opposite. The last check would be to re-add both columns and then, if there is still a discrepancy, look for a misread number—sometimes a one is entered for a seven or a three or five may have been carelessly entered.

Sometimes you may offer specials on services or products and might wonder how to enter those transactions. You ignore the discount and enter the amount actually paid. You would do the same if you received a discount on an item purchased from a supplier.

You may need to set up special journals, such as a cash receipts journal or a cash payments journal. Check with your accountant.

To make financial reports for your accounting period, you will have to make adjustments in your trial balance figures to allow for situations not recorded in your day-to-day entries and postings. For example, if you have not noted every change in your inventory that is a result of shoplifting, you will need to do so by making an inventory count and adjusting the account balance accordingly. Depreciation on equipment is another example of an adjustment needed for your capital asset account. You may owe wages that have not yet appeared on expense accounts because they have not yet been paid. There may be some charges that can never be collected. The book needs to know so that it will balance. All of these situations can be taken care of with the worksheet, an informal tool that is extremely useful.

A typical worksheet has ten columns, with a credit and debit column for each of five categories—unadjusted trial balance, adjustments, adjusted trial balance, income (operating) statement, and balance sheet.

Columns one and two are the unadjusted trial balance, which is achieved by simply copying the trial balance data into these columns. Some of the balances shown will be incorrect because adjustments have yet to be made, which is why this is called the "unadjusted" trial balance.

Columns three and four are where adjustments to the trial balance are entered. For example, if you began the accounting period with $150 worth of shopping bags and through inventory determined you were down to $35 worth of bags, you would know that $115 worth of bags had been used. You know now that your trial balance must be adjusted to reflect this usage.

When all the adjustments have been made, you extend the totals to arrive at your adjusted trial balance in columns five and six. If no adjustment was necessary for a particular account, you just bring the amounts from columns one and two over into five and six but, if there is a credit in column one and a debit in column four, you have to subtract one from the other and enter the result, whether a debit or credit, in column five or six. If column two and column four both show credits, these need to be added and the total carried into column six. If there is a debit in column one and an adjustment debit in column three, these are added and the sum put into column five. If done properly, columns three and four should be equal, as should columns five and six.

Columns seven and eight give you the operating statement. Line by line, choose only revenue and expense items from your adjusted trial balances (columns five and six) and enter them in seven and eight depending on whether they are debits or credits. Revenue accounts usually have credit balances. Expense items usually have debit balances.

Now that you have transferred all revenue and expense items to seven and eight, the remaining items will pertain to assets, liabilities, and capital and represent the data used in preparing the balance sheet. These items will consist of cash, accounts receivable, supplies, furniture and fixtures, machinery, land and buildings, and other property. These will be seen as a debit, recorded in column nine. Accumulated depreciation is known as a contra asset, as it is applied against capital assets, and is entered as a credit in column ten. Liability accounts such as salaries payable usually have credit balances and are put in column ten. The difference between columns seven and eight should be equal to the differences between nine and ten.

Part of the standardized format used in bookkeeping consists of dollar sign rules. These are: (1) Place a dollar sign at the top of each column representing money, and (2) Use a dollar sign after every addition or subtraction, that is, next to every total or result representing money.

FINANCIAL STATEMENTS

Now you are ready to prepare financial statements. By the way, there are other methods of keeping the books—this is just the method most commonly used. It bears repeating again, and maybe will make more sense after this brief look at bookkeeping: Consult with your accountant before setting up your system, and take a close look at computer systems, which can greatly reduce the time-consuming drudgery of the various bookkeeping tasks.

Two financial statements you'll want to produce are the operating statement and the balance sheet. You've already seen an example of an operating statement, or profit and loss statement. The balance sheet is compiled from columns nine and ten of the worksheet. While the operating statement uses the formula $R - E = NI$, the balance sheet must balance. Total assets must be the same as the totals of liabilities and capital.

The final step in the accounting cycle is to close the books. This readies them for the next accounting cycle.

If, as the owner, you work on a draw system for income, for each sum you draw, you credit cash and debit the drawing account. When closing, the debit balance in the drawing account is charged against capital.

After you have journalized every adjusting entry from columns three and four, a new T account called the account summary is created to summarize the data from all revenue and expense accounts. The closing process consists of these steps:

1. Bring revenue accounts to zero. Debit each revenue account in the ledger in the amount of its balance, which brings the accounts to zero and therefore ready to receive the next bookkeeping period's revenues. Then, you credit the income summary with the total of all revenues.
2. Bring expense accounts to zero by crediting each expense account in the amount of its balance. Debit the income summary by the total of all expenses.
3. Balance the income summary and adjust the capital account. Find the balance in the income summary account by adding the debit and the credit. If there is a profit, you will have a credit balance. You debit the income summary by this amount and credit the capital account. A minus balance in the income summary shows a business loss—credit the income summary for that amount and debit the capital account.
4. Adjust the owner's draw by crediting the drawing account in the amount of its balance and debiting the capital account in the same amount.

The last thing to do is to make journal entries for each step.

One last word about errors. They do occur, so a pencil is always recommended. Be careful of too many erasures—they may make your documents appear "doctored." Instead, draw a neat, single, ruled line through the wrong figure and write the correct figure above it. This clearly shows to any inquiring minds, such as the IRS, why the number was changed.

THE BENEFITS OF A PROPER ACCOUNTING AND BOOKKEEPING SYSTEM

The nine leading causes of business failure are lack of experience, insufficient inventory turnover, lack of business records, excessive accounts receivable, poor inventory control, improper markup, inadequate financing, inventory shrinkage (theft), and lack of sales. Eight of these can be managed through the proper accounting and bookkeeping system.

No matter what bookkeeping system you opt for, minimum requirements must be met. It must keep records in an orderly way, thus enabling you to know your accounts payable, cash on hand, accounts receivable, average sales, on-hand inventory, and profits. Next, it has to ensure proper tax planning. Then, it has to allow for proper records filing and retention, thereby allowing you to review what the salon has done in the past and reasonably predict what it will do in the future, essentials for cash flow management, obtaining credit, and planning for growth.

Whatever the system, it will be composed of four elements—the assets, the liabilities, the income, and the expenses. The system can be simple or complex. You can use a handwritten manual system of your own devising or one already designed, such as the one shown in this chapter, or you can use a computerized system. The important thing is to be sure the system is accurate, current, and provides you with all the information needed to run your business properly. Again, work closely with your accountant to set up the system best suited for your salon and to be sure you are making entries correctly and understand whatever bookkeeping system you elect to use. My own experience has been that the new technology available in software packages such as QuickBooks is far easier, quicker, and more accurate than posting debits and credits manually. As a person who has had a lifetime battle with any form of mathematics and accounting systems, a good software program has saved the day! There are several such programs available and the cost is relatively small, usually obtainable (the software, not the computer!) for under $200. If you can get around in a checkbook register, you can get around just as easily in many of the current accounting programs.

REVIEW

Bookkeeping is the method of keeping score for a business—a method of keeping track of the money that changes hands in the salon. Even if you perform most bookkeeping chores yourself, use an accountant to at least set up the system and monitor it.

The double-entry method of bookkeeping is the easiest to learn and probably the best for your salon. Whatever system is used, it should meet minimum requirements: it should keep records in an orderly way, ensure proper tax planning, and allow for proper records filing and retention. It should be accurate, current, and provide you with the information you need to run your business properly.

BUDGETING

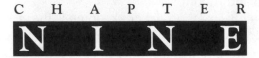

CHAPTER
NINE

Operating your salon at a profit is a constant challenge and a never-ending job. The primary requirement of a successful salon is that it earn a profit; a simple statement but one that bears repeating. Everything a salon owner does must be geared toward creating a profit for the business.

Proper pricing of services and products is crucial to profitability. Budgeting your expenses will help greatly in achieving a bottom line that is in the black, not the red, by allocating your available funds for their best possible use and by helping determine the proper pricing of your products.

The salon owner should do some research (using the budget as a primary tool) at least every six months to determine the pricing rates in your marketplace. By marketplace, I do not mean your geographical location, but the economic niche in which you have positioned yourself or are striving for.

Pricing services to return a profit is much more difficult than pricing retail products. Some basic factors to consider are:

- Shop the competition. Again, this doesn't mean those salons in your vicinity—it refers to salons competing in your perceived market.
- Analyze your competitors' pay scales in relation to their prices. It may well be that your competitor is paying excessive wages the

pricing structure doesn't support—possibly that salon is subsidized by outside income, for instance, a wife or husband's income from another source. In that case, you cannot reasonably expect to compete using their price ranges unless you have the same source of outside funding.

- Determine an overall price range and pay scale according to your expected business mix. Most salons pay a retail commission on products sold. Many separate such income from service income. You might want to look at ways to incorporate the two so that the stylist sees and understands that both are a necessary source of his or her income.
- From the information thus gathered, prepare an operating budget, based upon your anticipated sales figures and your expenses. Much of this information may be taken directly from the business plan you prepared earlier (see chapter 2).

Budgets will help you assess sales in both services and retail products; make week-to-week, month-to-month, year-to-year, and year-to-date comparisons of business activity; and tell you which stylist is performing and at what level for the salon.

SALARIES

A major expense in any salon budget will be salaries for stylists and other personnel, so it is imperative that you arrive at an equitable pay scale that is fair to both you and your employees. The first requirement must be that salaries paid do not wipe out profits—the business of business is to gain clients, keep them, and return a profit. Providing jobs for stylists is not the primary business of salons. In determining pay rates and scales, consult your accountant, and include several factors in any payroll determinations. One very important component is the tax/burden rate, which must be factored in if you are to have a realistic pay rate. The tax/burden rate is composed of the following items:

- FICA
- State Unemployment
- Federal Unemployment
- Workers' Compensation Insurance

Each state has its own unemployment and workers' comp rates, but for purposes of explanation, we will use the states of Indiana and Ohio.

TAX/BURDEN RATES

	Indiana Technical	Ohio Technical
FICA	7.6500%	7.6500%
State Unemployment	2.7000%	3.0000%
Federal Unemployment	0.8000%	0.8000%
Workers' Comp. Ins.	0.2709%	0.8646%
Total Burden Rate	11.4209%	12.3146%

This tells you, that you, as the employer, will have to pay this percentage of the employee's salary in various taxes. Put another way, if you pay an employee in Indiana $100.00 in wages, you will have actually paid out $111.43 ($100.00 x 11.4209%).

Then, you must determine how much you are going to pay the employee and how—either by salary, commission, or a combination of salary/commission or bonuses. Again, your accountant can help you figure a profitable and equitable rate and method of payment, factoring other employee expenses and overhead expenses into your calculations. Once you have figured the pay rate, you must figure what that person should charge for his or her services so that you both achieve your goals—the employee a reasonable salary for the work and you a reasonable profit on the labor.

FORECASTING THE FUTURE

Any business is continually faced with uncertainty about the future. This is the ultimate value of a budget—to better forecast that future based on past performance and informed estimates of cost and revenue trends. Forecasts such as employee hires, expansion, and adding products or services depend on your ability to be accurate in your prognostications.

Cost-volume-profit relationships are dependent upon accurate cost behavior descriptions. The interrelationships of all the affecting factors must be studied. For instance, you may want to add a new product line your supplier is ecstatic about, but before you go out on a limb and plunge

$3,000 into the line and that fantastic display case that comes with it, you need to know if you can reasonably expect to make a profit with it. You need to know how much advertising will be necessary to move the product, how much commission will be paid, how much physical space will be allocated to the product, the cost of the space, and all the other factors.

Any analysis must be made with regard to its limitations, essential in determining what a cost will be at a certain point (sales volume). Otherwise, you will not be able to regulate your costs properly, which is vital for efficient budgeting or forecasting.

Three types of costs must be part of your budget. Costs that remain the same over a period of time are referred to as fixed costs. Examples are rents, property taxes and insurances, depreciation, and support personnel's and owner's salaries. Costs that vary directly with changes in volume of sales, whether service or product sales, are known as variable costs, examples being sales commissions on products sold and service commissions. A third type of costs are semivariable costs, which have traits similar to both fixed and variable costs, such as the portion of rent paid on the building while it is not open for business.

One of the purposes of a budget is to determine breakeven points, which is that point of output where total revenues and total costs are equal. Controlling costs accurately depends on the ability of the owner or manager to forecast the effect on the breakeven point. To do this, the owner must continually analyze cost behavior and update breakeven points at regular intervals. The advent of the computer into the salon has made creating extremely helpful breakeven charts easier. If the program you are contemplating purchasing doesn't already have the ability to compile such charts, ask the company if it is possible to add this to the program and how easy or difficult it would be to do so. If you cannot obtain a program that will do this, your accountant may be able to help you devise longhand methods.

When determining profitability of a service such as a haircut or a permanent wave, or the retailing of a bottle of shampoo, the breakeven point must be known so that each may be priced correctly. The variable cost is the most important determinant, because from that the variable cost ratio (total variable costs divided by total sales) can be found, and once that ratio is determined, the total variable costs at any level of sales can be determined.

The contribution margin is the portion of the sales dollar available to cover fixed costs and attain a profit. It is arrived at by compiling variable costs and is computed by subtracting variable costs from sales. Future profits can be easily figured when the contribution margin is presented as a ratio of sales, and you can quickly see if the addition of a new line will be profitable, knowing the salon's ability to sell a certain amount of that product.

Here's how it works. Let's say you only do haircuts (for the sake of simplicity) and you price them at $20. You have determined your variable costs for a haircut are $12 per haircut. Your fixed costs (for a year) are $40,000. If you wish to earn a net gain of $24,000 for the year, the salon must perform 8,000 haircuts in the year. Can you see how important cost behavior patterns become?

These may seem like complicated formulas and data too difficult to arrive at. They really aren't—your accountant can explain just how easy it is to arrive at cost accounting and determine what it will take to earn a profit and how much. And it may be difficult, but it is a necessary part of business. The days are just about over when a stylist with a good following could just jump in and open a shop and hope everything turned up roses. It takes good business skills today to make success happen.

Getting back to our example, let's say you determine through market research that if you were to provide $10,000 worth of television advertising, you would be able to fill everyone's book currently working in the salon, which would mean an additional two thousand haircuts for the year. Net income would increase to $30,000, provided the cost and revenue estimates are accurate. Sometimes, profits may increase in a short-run situation but over the long haul suffer because your percentage margin is too low.

A good method of planning is to determine the profit goal you would realistically like to achieve. That figure plus the expected fixed costs will equal the contribution margin needed to cover the fixed costs and the desired profit. By figuring the expected operating volume, gross profit per haircut or other service can then be figured. Adding the expected variable cost per service to the gross profit will determine the net haircut sales figure that must be reached.

COSTS

Cost questions must be continually asked and reasked. Can they be changed? Can they be eliminated or reduced? Proper evaluation of costs allows you to take corrective action when necessary. For example, if you are paying your stylists too high a commission percentage to earn a satisfactory profit, you will see the problem and take steps to correct it, probably by lowering percentages.

If you have some misguided idea that commission percentages are sacred, you must be fairly new in the business! When I began styling hair in the mid-sixties, commissions paid to the stylist averaged 75 percent. I have even worked in salons where I was paid 85 percent! Now, some salons are paying as low as 35 percent. So, don't think that the commissions you are used to are somehow holy and untouchable. If you pay a commission rate that loses you money, you will have to change it or close your doors—it's that simple.

Cutting commissions is the last resort, however, when you have determined costs are too high. There are many other areas to investigate. Supply costs, for example. Enlist the aid of your staff by explaining to them just how important it is to both you and them to keep costs to a minimum. Cutting back on waste of shampoos, color products, and all the products used in servicing clientele will usually contribute to dramatic improvements in costs.

Maximizing resources is another way to cut costs. For instance, paying your receptionist, salon coordinator, or extra assistant to take care of day-to-day cleaning chores is an easily eliminated expense. Require that everyone in your salon do their part in emptying ashtrays, arranging magazines, and all the other little housekeeping duties as they see the need. Chances are you can drastically cut down the time spent by the receptionist or other person on this low-level activity and use his or her time for more productive jobs. This is a good example of paring costs.

You know your salon better than anyone else. Look at other ways of maximizing resources. Perhaps you offer a foil highlighting service and the stylist can opt to use either aluminum foil or plastic wrap. If plastic wrap is substantially less expensive (it is!), require all your stylists to use it, provided, of course, that the result is the same or better.

Keep an eye on each employee's use of supplies, such as shampoos and conditioners at the shampoo area. If you notice excessive use of products, have a private talk with the miscreant, explaining why it is important to be frugal. Show him or her ways to cut down and maintain the same high quality of service.

Your accountant, as you may be weary of noting, is your best source to set up a good working budget for your needs. After you arrive at a model to use, you must still work to perfect the instrument, constantly fine-tuning your budget until it is as good as it can be. (See Appendix B for some good references.)

Again, computers are especially valuable. Paper-and-pencil budgets are fast becoming a Dickensian artifact, and take up enormous amounts of time just as bookkeeping without a software program does. Those long hours spent toiling over a green sheet late at night can be cut virtually to nothing with the proper computer program. Stylists planning to open their first salon should think long and hard about computerizing—and then do it! The under $2,000 you will spend for the entire system will pay for itself over and over. Just ask anyone who has done it both ways.

REVIEW

A budget will help you assess sales of both services and retail products by making comparisons of business activities. The value of a budget is to better forecast the future based on past performance and informed estimates of cost and revenue trends.

A good method of planning is to determine your profit goals, add your fixed costs, and find your contribution margin, which is what you will need to achieve to make the desired profit. Computers can simplify the budget development process.

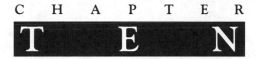

C H A P T E R
TEN

According to *The Random House College Dictionary,* Rev. Ed., two definitions for the word *husbandry* are: "3. careful or thrifty management." and, "4. the management of domestic affairs or of resources generally." That is what this brief chapter is about—the thrifty management of your resources.

MONEY IS A COMMODITY

First, be aware that money is a commodity, just like any other goods or services, and because it is a commodity, it has a value and a cost. When this particular commodity (money) lies idle, it is losing value because of various factors that influence it, such as inflation. If you had $100 ten years ago and hid it under your mattress, and inflation had occurred at the average rate of 5 percent each year, you would have lost 50 percent of its buying power in that period. If you had invested it in a savings instrument that paid an average of 10 percent per year, your $100 would have grown faster than inflation and be worth much more. This is fairly straightforward and doesn't figure out exactly as depicted, but you get the picture. Money lying idle is losing value. (Figure 10.1)

FIGURE 10.1
Money lying idle is losing value. Make your bank your financial partner.

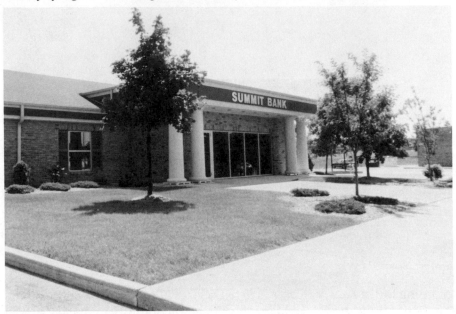

USE CASH-ON-HAND TO GENERATE INCOME

The same thing happens when you don't use your cash-on-hand to generate income. There are a hundred ways in which this happens in the average salon. For instance, you buy six dozen perms and the dealer allows you two paying options—to pay cash upon delivery or to pay the same amount in ninety days without penalty, interest, or extra charge. Many would pay cash, but a more aware salon owner would take advantage of the ninety days, and pay at the last possible moment. The owner exercising the second option will earn money on his or her money in two ways if the amount is kept in an interest-bearing instrument, such as a money market or savings account or a checking account that pays interest. First, he or she will pay off the debt with inflated dollars, saving money. Inflation in today's society is a given—it is relatively safe to say that the dollar you have in your hand today is not going to have the same value (purchasing power) in even as short a period as ninety days. The value of the goods (perms) purchased has stayed the same, or perhaps even risen, and now the owner is paying it off with money that is worth less. By placing the money representing the cost of the perms in an instrument (such as an interest-bearing checking account) that pays interest (earns money), the owner has also earned income on the use of the money. He or she has done what is called "using the float." Most astute business people always use the float, i.e., they take full advantage of the grace period for all bills. It is a commonly accepted practice and there is nothing unethical or illegal about it whatsoever, as some persons mistakenly seem to think. Ask your product dealers if they use the float with their accounts payable, and if they are forthright, I will bet a large sum that they will admit to doing so as a common practice. If you are not taking advantage of the float, you should be doing so.

Bear two things in mind when using the float. Don't go past the grace period (thirty, sixty, and ninety days are usual) and end up paying penalties and/or interest, or you have defeated the purpose and will probably end up losing money. And don't just let the money sit, not earning interest or at least being utilized for other payables that will reduce an interest load.

Years ago, I sold life insurance for Prudential, and sometimes we advised the client to purchase term insurance in lieu of whole life, and use the difference in premiums to invest. The interest paid on whole life is usually substantially less than would be earned in even a basic bank savings account. Clients who did so realized a significant return; those who chose to just spend the money lost a large sum over the years. The point is, put the money you would have spent on the perms to work until it is time to pay it and you will be practicing good husbandry.

Using the float amounts to an interest-free loan. If you use this loan to create additional wealth, you have used it wisely. If you don't invest wisely, you'll still have the loan (perm bill) to pay off!

Again, ask your bank and your accountant for the best means of investing this money. Shop around. Each bank or banking chain has different options. Most interest-bearing checking accounts have minimum balances that must be maintained before they will earn interest, but some banks have lower balances than others, or they may pay higher rates with different accounts. Always remember to compare apples to apples, never apples to oranges, and get advice from your accountant.

Hark back to chapter 8, and don't get into crisis management at the end of the year when you're trying to figure out where to put taxable money to avoid Uncle Sam's bite. This is another form of resource husbandry that you should be aware of and prepare for with your financial advisor or accountant.

REVIEW

Resource husbandry is very simple. Use your money, don't let it lie around doing nothing and being consumed by inflation. Remember these simple rules:

1. Buy now.
2. Pay later, with inflated dollars.
3. Invest the money you would have spent.
4. Congratulate yourself for being shrewder than your competition!

EQUIPMENT PURCHASES

C H A P T E R
ELEVEN

"There is more than one way to skin a cat," goes the old saying, and that old saw is especially true when it comes to not only designing your salon, but picking out the equipment, and even paying for it.

There are many creative floor plans, perhaps as many different plans as there are salons. Local equipment distributors are the logical source for most designing needs, but don't overlook firms in your area that design office space for other types of small businesses. Such firms may be able to come up with unique ideas not thought of by your local or even national distributors. The advantage of this kind of design company is that they will probably be dealing with a business (hair salon) with which they are not familiar. Instead of this being a disadvantage, it can be a plus, in that they will be looking at it with fresh eyes and may be able to arrive at designs and layouts salon design professionals would not see.

However, design firms that are not specifically in the salon design business may be unaware of regulations concerning space requirements and other licensing and regulatory laws. For instance, the National Cosmetology Association recommends 130 to 150 square feet of space for each cosmetologist, and it (NCA) advises checking with your state board of cosmetology for additional requirements. There also may be hot water regulations, sanitary laws, and other salon requirements.

There may be other disadvantages to selecting such a company to design your salon. Traffic pattern flows, for instance, may be misinterpreted, resulting in a salon that doesn't provide for maximum efficiency. Also, most distributors and equipment companies provide a design service free of charge, while an independent designer most certainly won't! In fact, their charges are usually quite high, and only advisable for very high-end salons, and even those kinds of salons can do very nicely with the services offered by local supply houses, distributors, and equipment manufacturers. And, although such services are given free or for a very nominal charge, there is nothing second class about the product they provide.

Plus, they know the business. That factor cannot be underestimated. A large, national equipment manufacturer that has been in business for a long time has weeded out floor designs that are inefficient or unattractive and, with its vast store of knowledge, can design a salon based on virtually any size and dimensions and for almost any budget.

Another designer source is students at local colleges or trade and technical schools that offer architectural design in one form or another. Often, a school with design programs will have students who are eager for practical experience in design or in perfecting their CAD-CAM (Computer Aided Drawing) techniques, and will be glad to come in and create a layout for a very nominal fee or simply a class credit. Phone the educational institutions in your area to ascertain if such programs exist, then contact the person in charge of the program to see if there is a possibility of obtaining inexpensive or free design aid for your salon.

Remember that whoever designs your salon must be aware of the legal requirements pertaining to electrical and plumbing codes, as well as cosmetology law requirements—and there may be laws in your state that prohibit or restrict such efforts except from licensed contractors or firms.

One more design source is yourself. If the salon is to be relatively small and simple, perhaps you are the best person to create the floor plan. It is certain that no one else will have more of an interest than you will! For the computer hackers, design programs are available to assist you if you have the time and expertise to enable you to use them. Such programs are mostly ultra-sophisticated and eat up lots of memory on computers, so it is not the best idea to run out and purchase such a program unless you are really computer savvy. If you do decide to do your own planning, it may be a good idea to at least run the finished schematic by a reputable dealer that provides design service for an opinion. They may well be able to point out flaws you haven't seen or prepared for, and may be able to give you suggestions that will make the plan an even better one. Almost always, such advice is free, assuming, of course, that you plan on purchasing some of your equipment and supplies from them.

A number of floor plans have been furnished by the Belvedere Company, long-time makers of salon equipment and furniture. (Figures 11.1 through 11.5) A good sample of various layouts is included, to at least give you an idea of what may be accomplished for your space. Belvedere, as well as any equipment manufacturer, has people on staff who do nothing but design salons for clients, normally a free service. You may contact them through your local outlet or at the address and phone number listed in Appendix B.

FIGURE 11.1
Salon floor plan. *Courtesy Belvedere Equipment Company, Inc.*

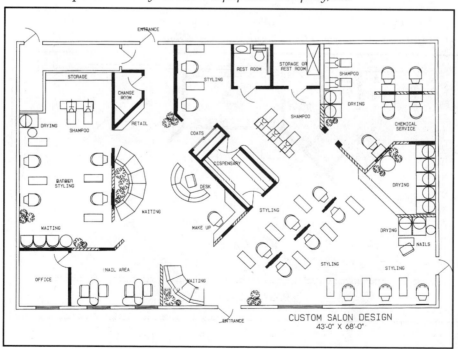

CUSTOM SALON DESIGN
43'-0" X 68'-0"

FIGURE 11.2
Salon floor plan. *Courtesy Belvedere Equipment Company, Inc.*

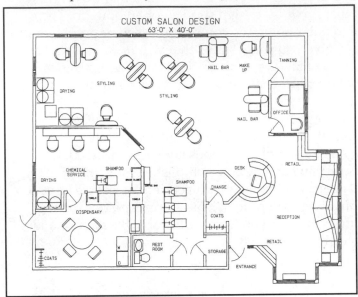

FIGURE 11.3
Salon floor plan. *Courtesy Belvedere Equipment Company, Inc.*

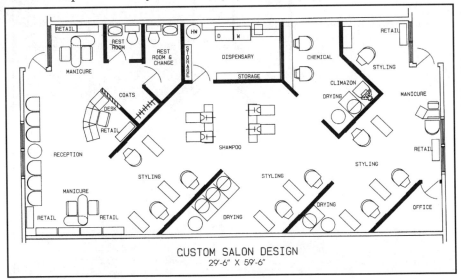

FIGURE 11.4
Salon floor plan. *Courtesy Belvedere Equipment Company, Inc.*

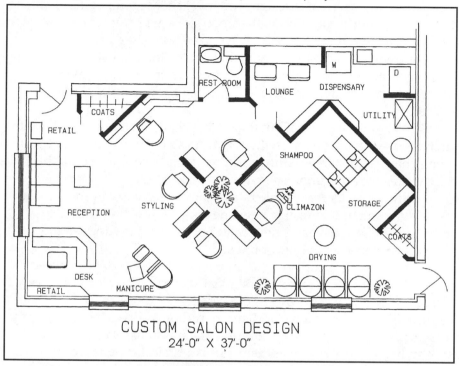

FIGURE 11.5
Salon floor plan. *Courtesy Belvedere Equipment Company, Inc.*

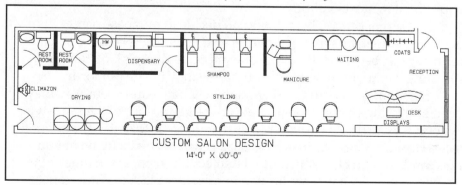

CHOOSING EQUIPMENT

Once you have arrived at a design, you must choose your equipment. Much of the equipment, such as shampoo sinks, will have to be of a standard nature and will probably have to be purchased at a beauty or barber supply outlet. Perhaps you will want to obtain most of your equipment through such standard vendors. For those with a more adventuresome nature, and who love a bargain, other options are available.

For example, instead of buying styling chairs new, you may wish to purchase used chairs and have them reupholstered inexpensively. Most styling chairs are relatively sturdy and of a simple design, and all that really wears out is the upholstery. If you can locate an upholsterer who does quality work for reasonable rates, many times you can end up with a chair that can't be told from a new one at two thirds the cost. And remember, when you bring a new chair home from the supplier and sit in it that chair is no longer new but used.

Often the same supplier who carries new lines also takes in used equipment on trade-ins and has just what you're looking for in the back room. Bob Van Cleave, the owner of Professional Hair Designers Products (PHD) of Ft. Wayne, Indiana, a leading Midwest beauty supply house, says he gets many such equipment items in regularly and has a list of stylists eagerly awaiting them. His is a typical experience, he says, among supply house owners, as many hair stylists see the value in refurbishing older equipment, ending up with a piece of furniture that looks new for a fraction of the cost. By far, PHD sells and leases more new than used equipment, but there is a source and a market for used equipment in most localities.

A word of caution here. If you do decide to purchase part of your equipment used, be sure you have located someone who can do quality refurbishing, because if the piece of equipment doesn't look first-rate, the money you save won't be worth the shabby image put forth.

Sometimes you can't find enough matching equipment. You may need six styling chairs but can locate only three or four of the same type. A good way to obtain enough pieces that match is to watch the paper for salon closings. Chances are a single salon will have exactly what you need and enough of it. Watch the classified ads in papers in other cities as well, especially if you are located in a smaller market. For instance, here in Ft. Wayne, I would look at papers from Chicago, Cleveland,

Detroit, St. Louis, and Indianapolis, if I needed a large number of styling chairs. Each of those cities is within a two- or three-hour drive from where I am, and it is certainly worth the drive if I can locate something inexpensive enough. If you are unable to obtain newspapers from towns not in your immediate vicinity, most libraries carry them.

One of New Orleans' top salons, Busta at the Fairmont, had a novel idea for styling chairs when I worked there. Busta used specially designed canvas captain's chairs that looked great and were one of the easiest chairs to work with you could ever imagine. He had two sizes of chairs, and the stylist would choose the appropriate chair depending upon the height of the client. The chairs alone set the salon apart from most others, and clients were impressed with the comfort as well as the unusual look. Another advantage was that, with the relatively low price of the chairs, they could be changed every year or so, giving the salon the look of a major redecoration for a small outlay.

Years ago, I put in a salon on a limited budget and was able to design a very distinctive-looking salon for a very small amount. I decided on a rustic decor. Driving through the countryside, I saw a family in the process of tearing down an old barn. They were glad to give me any of the wood I wanted simply for hauling it away. Out of the handpicked load, I was able to find some wonderful old wood with which I fashioned backbar shelving upon which to hang tools and display products, solving the problem of a backbar unit. Above these simple shelves, I hung mirrors framed with the same wood. At a railroad salvage company, I found, among other useful items, brand-new wooden nail kegs for a quarter apiece. Six of the kegs, filled with white sand, provided very attractive, eye-catching product displayers. I obtained the mirrors for a pittance from a large department store that had filed bankruptcy. They were the long ones hung on columns, over fifteen feet long in some instances, and easy enough to cut into the shapes and sizes I wanted.

Waiting room furniture can be acquired in much the same way. Instead of purchasing new, look around at garage sales or used furniture outlets and you may be surprised at the buys available. Again, just be sure you have a professional upholsterer who can do quality work at a good price if you go that route.

And steal ideas! If you see a great look outside of your market area that you think you could duplicate inexpensively, do it! As far as I know, salon layouts cannot be copyrighted, so I doubt if you'll have to worry about a lawsuit if you copy Salon Z's decor, especially if Salon Z is located three states away. And, isn't imitation the sincerest form of flattery?

PAYING FOR EQUIPMENT

Now, how to pay for it! The equipment and furnishings you get from supply houses can be financed in a variety of ways. The old-fashioned method of cash on the barrelhead still works—most people won't turn down hard currency—but it may be in your best interest to finance your operation another way.

Leasing options abound, and most suppliers and equipment companies have several plans from which to choose. Bob Van Cleave, of the aforementioned PHD supply house, has a variety of plans, including one they use with Kimco Leasing, Inc. called the 12+1 Program. This is a very simple plan, as most leasing programs are. Its features are:

- Customer's (purchasing salon) payment = cost divided by twelve
- Thirteen payments
- $1 Buy-out option
- $795 Minimum

If the equipment you want to purchase will cost, say, $12,000, then that amount is divided by twelve, which equals $1,000, and the loan is paid back in thirteen equal monthly payments of $1,000 each. The cost of the loan would therefore be $1,000, which figures out to around $8\,1/2$ percent interest. At the end of the payment period, the salon owner then purchases the equipment for $1. PHD uses this method quite a bit, making it, in Bob Van Cleave's own words, "about the same and as easy as buying a used car."

In this leasing example, the salon owner gets a very advantageous loan rate and his or her money isn't tied up in equipment, freeing that amount for other things. Usually there is no down payment required, and leasing programs basically allow you to use the equipment and pay for it as it helps you create income, letting the equipment, in effect, pay for itself.

This is by no means the only lease plan. Equipment can be financed or leased in literally dozens of ways, and most good suppliers will be glad to work with you and your budget to get you the best deal.

If you would like to look into leasing and none of your suppliers seems to be set up for any programs, look in your yellow pages under Leasing, and chances are good that a company will be listed that can create a program for you. Normal credit requirements, such as a good credit history and perhaps some collateral, apply in most cases, although when leasing arrangements are made through a local supplier, many times the supplier's knowledge of your character and ability may offset weaker credit histories.

According to Century Financial Services Group, Ltd. (CFS), 15455 Conway Road, Suite 350, Chesterfield, Missouri 63017, leasing can provide the following advantages:

- Prompt credit approvals.
- Fixed rate financing.
- Terms up to sixty months.
- Finance 100 percent of equipment cost.
- No down payment required.
- Maximizes tax benefits.
- Conserves bank credit lines and conserves cash.
- You are acquiring equipment today and paying for it with tomorrow's cheaper dollars (inflation).
- Maintains financing flexibility.
- Eliminates the traditional lengthy credit approval process.

CFS, one of the largest leasing companies working in the salon field, like many such leasing entities, will finance 100 percent of the equipment costs, taxes, installation, and delivery charges, which allows for minimum up-front cash requirements. They say that "ownership of equipment alone will *not* produce revenue. It is the *use* of equipment that is productive. When viewed from this perspective, leasing is frequently less expensive."

The venerable equipment company, Belvedere, maintains that "a lot of salon people are so married to the conventional methods of financing equipment, they never look at how leasing can get them more of their dream than they ever dreamed possible." Belvedere provides a comparison chart between leasing and outright purchase. (Table 11.1)

Most experts today advise to lease if possible, but it is always best to check with your accountant before you make a decision. Tax laws that might be favorable to leasing situations at this writing may change by

TABLE 11.1

	Leasing	Financing
Term	Up to 5 years on any system	Usually 2–3 yrs.
Down Pymt.	Usually 1st & last month's lease pymt.	Typically 20–30%
Int. Rate	Fixed rate	Usually floating rate, customer takes all the risks
Hidden Chgs.	None	Compensating balances & other charges, loan covenants
Tax Benefits	Usually 100% deductible; makes effective cost lower	Can only deduct depreciation of equip. over 5 yrs. (15% 1st yr); principle not deductible.
Effective Cost	Lower than prime rate due to tax advantages, length of lease, and no down payment	Higher than published interest rate due to hidden costs

the time you start to plan your salon, and your financial advisor or accountant may be able to show you a better way to go. Or, if leasing is still the most advantageous, your accountant may be able to direct you to the best leasing situation. Many companies will customize plans to fit your needs, budget, and plans.

COMPUTERS IN THE SALON

One piece of equipment that a few short years ago was thought to be a luxury item reserved only for the most upscale of salons or the large operations, but now considered almost a necessity for even the smallest of salons, is the computer.

We are not going to get into a detailed analysis of what kind of system you should buy, or even if you should become computerized at all, except to provide a general overview and point out that time is money. The right computer set-up can save the average salon owner enormous amounts of time in bookkeeping, budgeting, payroll records, mailings, client files, inventory control and tracking, marketing, and management of the salon. There are dozens of ways the computer is utilized in today's salon. (Figure 11.6)

FIGURE 11.6
The computer can even be used to design the salon, using one of the space-designing programs available.

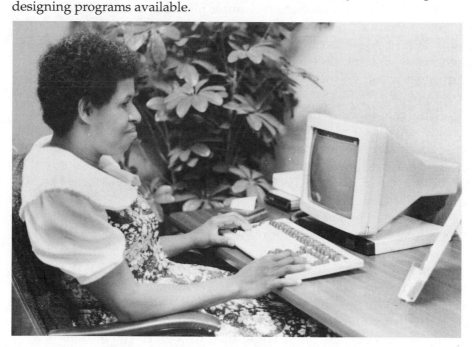

When computers first came out, a number of companies offered salon packages and programs, many of which were legitimate and worth the money, but many of which were oversold and overpriced. As salon owners became more aware and knowledgeable about computers and programs, spurious kinds of snake-oil salespeople have declined in number, although a few are still out there, so beware and deal only with those you can trust.

As computer technology changes almost minute by minute, any textbook runs the risk of being out-of-date almost by the time it comes from the printer, before it even gets in your hands. Don't be intimidated by the technology—it is far simpler than you would imagine and easy for anyone to master.

We have a saying in our salon, that if the computer goes on the fritz, or we run into a problem, we run out and find the first twelve-year-old we can—they'll know what to do! That is truer than you think—most kids are already learning about computers in the early elementary grades. If a small child can operate them (and they can!) then an adult capable of establishing and running a small business like a hairstyling salon should have no problems whatsoever.

For those of you who are computer illiterate, don't feel bad—all of us were at one point. No one was born with a computer knowledge gene. There are some very simple things to be aware of. First, most systems have five main components. The hardware (the computer, the keyboard, the screen, and a printer) and a software program.

The computer itself contains a hard drive or floppy disks. Don't even consider anything less than a hard drive. Floppy disks are too inconvenient and don't have enough storage capacity for multiple applications. They are all right, perhaps, for single-use applications, such as word processing, but for the kinds of uses a salon has, they just won't work. Also, as far as I know, salon programs will only work on a hard drive.

The size of main memory in the hard drive is very important. There must be enough to support the program(s) and to store the information you will want to record. Minimum requirements are that the computer come with 650K RAM (main memory) and 20MB to 40MB hard disk, although that is becoming dated, as most computers today come with 80MB hard disk as standard main memory and much higher for very little extra cash outlay. More main memory allows you to run larger programs, and a larger hard disk gives you the ability to store more data.

And don't think that whatever you start out with is all you'll ever need. Who would have ever thought six or seven years ago that styling salons would be able to use programs that run telemarketing plans? Well, that day is here! A handful of salons right now have their computers dialing numbers and making sales pitches, obtaining market research, and performing other marketing functions over the phone, in the evening when the salon is closed and the owners are at home eating supper. At this writing there are but a few, but such innovations are the wave of the future, and if today's salon owners don't keep up with the technology, someone's going to eat their lunch.

Even the very smallest salon would probably benefit from computerizing. Maybe the smallest salon would actually benefit the most as, traditionally, the owner of a one- or two-chair salon puts in enormous hours doing the books, ordering, inventorying, and completing all the seemingly thousands of tasks that come with the territory. Computers can give you back enormous chunks of time, not to mention do most jobs more efficiently.

Look at what just one company's specially designed salon program can do. The following is lifted verbatim from Leprechaun Salon Software's marketing booklet:

LEPRECHAUN
Marketing/Management Features

Point of Sale:
- Automatic Client Look Up
- On-Screen Client Profiles
- Client First and Last Visit Dates
- Perm and Color Information
- Complete Client History
- Quick Client Check-out
- Automatic Pricing
- Line Item Discounts
- Split Payment Methods
- House Charges
- Fast End of Day Balancing
- Complete End of Day Reporting

Management:
- Daily Reports
- Salon Summaries
- Salon Productivity Reports
- Employee & Salon Evaluation Reports
- Comparative Sales Analysis
- Inventory Sales Tracking
- Cash Receipts & Disbursements
- Year to Year Comparisons
- Payroll Information
- Goals
- Password Protected

Marketing:
- Promotion & Retention Reports
- Advertising Analysis
- New Client Listing
- Over 100 Marketing Selections
- Client Mailing Labels
- Lost Client Reporting
- Client Reminders

Courtesy of Leprechaun Salon Software.

The Leprechaun salon program is offered at a very affordable price, and theirs is by no means the only such program. Many programs exist, and this is by no means an endorsement for only Leprechaun (addresses and phone numbers of it and other computer and software companies are listed in Appendix B), as there are many others that can do an excellent job for you. Or, if you are one of the gifted (the computer literate), you can perhaps adapt one of the hundreds of general programs that proliferate in the industry for your own use. Just be sure to choose a program that is user-friendly so that those in the salon who will be using it don't go around the bend trying to figure out how to run it!

If you are not familiar with computers in general, it would pay you to become so. Most colleges offer basic computer classes, as do many retail outlets. The only thing about retail stores and their classes is that they are naturally trying to sell you their product, which may not be the best purchase for your needs. As you learn more and more about the computing industry, you will see great disparities in prices, and you will begin to find outlets that are much cheaper than what you imagined. A fair amount of networking goes on in the computer world, and it can pay you to pick the brains of your clients who work with computers. Many times they are your best source of education and can steer you in the right direction.

Computers are now a commodity, and the best pricing is through discount stores and mail order companies. Your best bet is to consult with someone whose judgment and knowledge you trust, and then order from one of these outlets. The software program cited here, Leprechaun, is an example of a mail order product.

As in other equipment purchases, paying cash or setting up payment programs may not be as fiscally wise as investigating the benefits of leasing. You can get a whole lot more bang for your computing buck by leasing, get more "bells and whistles," and pay for it with inflated dollars, plus realize a substantial offset in taxes.

Also, many times we complain about junk mail, but if you want to teach yourself about computers, send for some of the free catalogues listed in computer magazines, and see how quickly your name is sold to other lists and you begin getting reams of computer-related mail! Rather than being a burden on your mailbox, these can be a source of good information, and many good buys and bargains abound once you know what to look for. Pick up some of the computer magazines at your local bookstore or magazine outlet; you can learn a lot from their articles and ads. Your local librarian should be able to recommend a good text or two that can at least familiarize you with the terms and jargon, and business supply houses can usually recommend good texts as well.

One pitfall to avoid with computers—they can become so darned much fun to play around with that you get very little else done! This sounds amusing, but it can be true. If you do computerize, make sure you don't neglect attending to salon business. It is easy to get so addicted to the computer screen and all the aforementioned bells and whistles that you kid yourself into thinking what you're doing is productive when it really isn't. Just keep in mind that a computer is just a tool—a very worthwhile and helpful tool, but a tool just the same as your styling chair is.

And price-wise, the trick with computers and related services and goods is to shop around. You will be amazed at the wide differences in prices on essentially the same piece of equipment. Here is a good example. Recently, I purchased a Hewlett-Packard DeskJet Printer and decided I wanted to expand the print style capability, which meant I had to purchase a font cartridge. I looked in our local yellow pages for stores that carried Hewlett-Packard and called one. What I was after cost $270. After I picked myself up off the floor, I politely thanked them and said I'd get back to them. I called Hewlett-Packard's toll-free number to ask them if they would sell the part directly to me, which they wouldn't (worth a try!). They did, however, give me the phone number of a store in a different state (that would mail me the part). I called this store in Michigan and was quoted a price of $70—for the same font!

With computers, as with all equipment, it pays to shop!

REVIEW

If you use a design firm that doesn't usually design salons, you get the advantage of a fresh outlook. Disadvantages are that they may not be familiar with salon needs and you may have to pay more for the design. Whoever designs the salon must be aware of legal requirements affecting it.

When you are purchasing equipment, think of creative ways to save money by purchasing used equipment, which you can have refurbished to look like new. You may decide to pay cash, but leasing has numerous advantages, the main one being that you can use your cash for other things.

Even the smallest salon can benefit from purchasing a computer, and this purchase is another good prospect for leasing.

C H A P T E R

TWELVE

"When you're ripe you're rotten—when you're green you're growing!" A hoary old saying with a lot of truth to it that is usually applied to the lifelong learning experience, but can be applied with accuracy to the building of a prosperous salon. There is an axiom in business that you must always be increasing the volume or fall by the wayside—again, an adage with more than a kernel of truth to it.

Not being properly prepared for growth can be disastrous. You must have sound financial plans to accommodate growth. Some signals will tell you when it is time to expand the salon.

One sure tip-off is when you are being swamped by demand. When you are losing clientele because you and your staff cannot fit them in, it is time for expansion. Or if you are accommodating clients, but it is requiring a superhuman effort to do so, it is time to add staff, make price changes, or both.

When you begin to hear requests from clients for services or products you don't offer or carry, it is time to look into the feasibility of providing those services or goods. (Figure 12.1) There is a twofold danger in not acting in such instances. If you choose not to add a requested line or service you will lose the revenue from that particular product or service, and the client will eventually find his or her way to an outlet that provides it. Chances are excellent that that outlet will also provide services or goods you currently furnish to the client, but for shopping ease, he or she will begin to purchase those items or services at that site as well.

FIGURE 12.1
"Look, I've had six requests just this week for sculptured nails. Are we going to offer them?" When you begin to get requests for services you don't carry, it may be time to carry them.

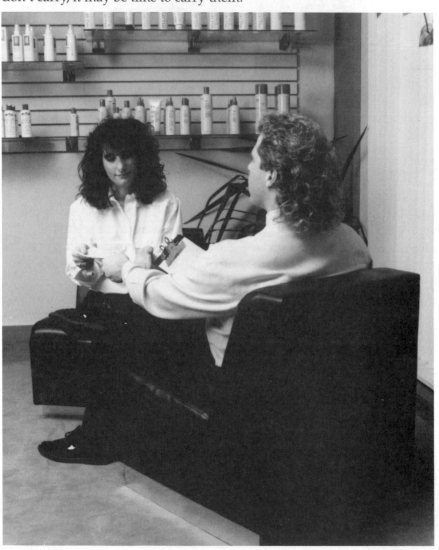

Example: You cut, perm, and highlight Brenda's hair, and she begins asking if you are going to be offering the service of sculptured nails. You have been getting quite a few requests for that service lately, but you have decided you don't want to enter the market, even though there seems to be a demand for it. You tell Brenda no, you're sorry, but you won't be offering any nail services of that kind. You may even recommend a place you know for the service. It doesn't matter if you do or don't—if she has a desire for sculptured nails she will find a place that will provide them for her. And once she has gone there for her nails, chances are excellent (if it is a salon setting) that they will eventually obtain her hair needs business as well. Getting someone to walk in the door is half the sales battle in our business. Remember that the next time you dismiss out of hand adding a new service or product, especially if that item has been heavily requested. You may be losing more than just the income from that service!

Another opportunity to expand comes about when you observe that you just have too few staff members to service existing clientele. You may not be losing clients, but they may be having to wait longer and longer for appointments. (Figure 12.2)

FIGURE 12.2
The rewards of hard work! When word of mouth has increased your business to where you can't handle the growing clientele, it's time to expand.

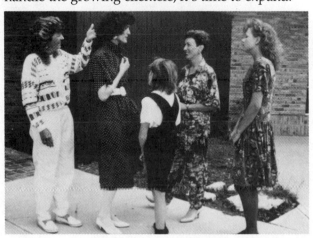

DIVERSIFICATION

Even though we are in the salon business, we can take a page from other businesses and think about diversification. Smart business owners watch for chances to expand in other directions and pounce when the opportunity arises. The more diversified you become, the less affected by sudden trends in the buying public you'll be. Expansion within the same general area still qualifies as diversification. For instance, you may have space available that isn't operating at a profit, and a small boutique would fit that spot nicely. You are providing a new and different product for an already existing clientele, and yet it is still within the general profile of the salon, which is fashion. History abounds with companies and businesses of all sorts that were heavily and singly into one exclusive product or service and got caught with their pants down when the market mood shifted. In our own industry this has happened time and time again. Older hands can tell you what happened to the shops and salons that depended entirely on a roller-set clientele—thirty years ago they were the norm, today they have all but disappeared, and even the ones left usually must offer more than just roller sets in order to keep their doors open. (Figure 12.3)

Years ago, the railroad companies were asked to make an investment in airplanes, but they said no thanks. They claimed they

FIGURE 12.3
Don't get caught sleeping when the market changes.

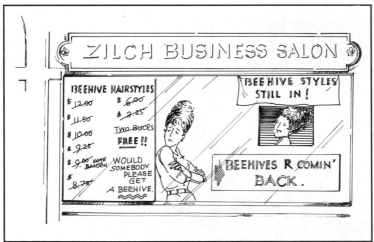

were in the train business and had no need for airplanes. The airline industry had approached the train companies because they assumed they were in the transportation business. Well, everyone knows what happened because of their (train companies') lack of foresight. Airlines have grown and prospered, while trains have seriously declined.

Diversification doesn't always have to be strictly along the lines of what the salon already offers. If you have an expertise in a given area and see a demand among existing clientele for that product or service, and you have made provision in your business plan for such opportunities, you may capitalize on an idea that may ultimately prove even more lucrative than the salon itself.

Some salons began serving refreshments to clients and got so good at it, they opened small cafes in conjunction with the salon. At our own salon, we have opened a small "remaindered" book store and are involved in setting up a mail order book business. We took space in the waiting area to set up a small book exhibit and the results have been outstanding. During the Christmas gift-buying season, we expect to sell a lot of merchandise.

The point is, when funds and opportunity become available, think about expanding the salon by either adding personnel, adding services or products, or diversifying.

FRANCHISING

Another method of quickly expanding your business is to franchise. There are many ways of setting up franchises, and it is advisable to check with recognized experts in the field before you venture forth. Your attorney should be able to guide you in the proper direction should franchising be an option you wish to investigate.

PROVIDING FOR CASH

Another factor in planning your growth is systematically providing for influxes of cash when needed. From the first day of business, you should be doing all you can to establish a positive credit rating. Initial credit for most salons is established through trade accounts with product dealers. As you comply with the account's terms, you begin to establish the credit worthiness of the salon. Then, as the salon matures, you will want to establish commercial credit. A line of credit or a business loan may become desirable or even necessary to carry out your plans or capitalize on an opportunity.

The best way to secure loans is to prepare far in advance. Send frequent operating statements to your lending institution—perhaps as often as monthly or quarterly at the very least. Lending institutions want to know if a requested loan is sufficient for the business needs, that it makes sense for the business, and that the loan will be repaid. Financial projections, which can be used to show the lender that you will need $7,000 now and $4,000 in six months, should be done in detail for at least three years. A good business plan can substantiate such a request and show the loan pay-off over the time period. Even more importantly, it prevents you from showing up at the bank each month asking for an additional $2,000, an approach that will hurt your credibility and put an unwelcome light on your ability to manage your business.

TAX PLANNING

Proper tax planning can help give you the capital needed for expansion. The three recognized methods of tax planning are transactional tax planning, strategic tax planning, and post year-end tax planning (more commonly and accurately known as "crisis management" and obviously the least desirable method).

Transactional tax planning concerns itself with the reduction of the tax consequence of a single event or series of events to its lowest total. Let's say you are considering selling all of your styling chairs so that you may purchase new ones. In transactional planning, you need to answer certain questions before you make the deal. For example, should the sale of the chairs be reported on the installment basis? Are the chairs depreciable or are they an investment asset? What is your tax bracket this year compared to subsequent years (estimation)? Is the sale to a related party? These pertinent questions will determine if selling the chairs is a wise move at this time.

Strategic tax planning is an ongoing program of when income should be recognized and when expenses ought to be paid. Usually, this is performed in the last months of the fiscal year, and the overall objective is to receive income in the year in which it will benefit from the lowest tax rate and to pay out expenses in the year in which they will best offset the highest tax. There are several techniques your accountant can advise you to use. Such techniques might involve prepayment of expenses or groupings of itemized deductions limited by percentages of adjusted gross income. To use strategic planning the most effectively, you have to estimate the current year's income as well as accurately foretell future years' income. Sound planning can give you a fairly accurate estimate.

The last and absolutely least effective way to manage and plan taxes is the method used by salons that don't take advantage of accounting wisdom and assistance—crisis management or post year-end tax planning. It is the least effective since once a transaction has been consummated, most planning opportunities are gone. Using this method of planning leaves very few options, limited mainly to decisions on how much to invest in a SEP or an IRA.

Tax laws change quickly and further complicate the ability to effectively plan tax deferral or avoidance if you utilize the latter method. A good tax planning program depends on working closely with a qualified accountant and investing the time to remain current on tax law changes, as well as obtaining a complete understanding of the effect of those laws on a selected tax avoidance plan. In other words, become a working partner with your accountant and if you are unfamiliar with tax planning, work to become educated.

Tax planning can help you provide necessary funds for future expansion, as well as demonstrate to any potential lender you have control of your business and are utilizing sound practices in its management. This can tip the decision your way when requesting loan funds.

Proper planning can lead to the fulfillment of some very extraordinary dreams, probably unachievable without such forethought. I once worked for an outstanding stylist and even better businessman who, with prudent planning, ended up owning a shopping center. His abilities, both in styling hair and in running a business, made his salon the number one in town. Many in the same position would have been content with what they had achieved, but not this man. He had bigger and better dreams. He decided he wanted his own building and, better yet, he wanted someone else to pay for it. Since he was already cutting the hair of many of the town's leading businessmen and women, he picked their brains, and came up with the idea of building a shopping center.

When he first approached a bank with his idea, they politely turned him down. Next, he applied for a Small Business Administration-guaranteed loan, but that, too, was denied. Did he give up? No. He knew he had a good idea and one that would work. His next step was ingenious. He acted as though he already had the funds and went out and solicited written promises from reputable business people to lease space in his shopping center before it had even been built—before he had even obtained the loan for building it! He even got the U.S. Postal Service to agree to lease space for a station, a very solid tenant-to-be for sure!

Armed with the promises of space leased at 100 percent, he got the bank to agree to loan him the money necessary to purchase the land and build the mall. Naturally, he took the prime anchor position for his own salon, and ended up not only getting his salon for literally nothing, but also creating enormous capital and income.

This is not to say every salon owner will be able to do what this man did—in fact, there are very few with the contacts to achieve what he did—but whatever your dreams or goals are, they will be virtually impossible to achieve without proper planning. This man's dream would have remained just that if he hadn't prepared himself by learning all there was to learn about taxes, business, and finance. There are those who decry such successes by saying the person was merely lucky, but my observation has been that luck is a funny gift—it seems to fall mostly on those who are prepared to receive it.

Proper planning is necessary to tell you if and when you should change your business structure. For example, there are three basic business structures—sole proprietorships, partnerships, and corporations. Based on the laws at this writing, taxes paid on income below $60,000 a year are less for a sole proprietor or partner than for a corporation; above $60,000, taxes are lower for a corporation. (Note: This is true at this writing—the law may change by the time you read this to favor one or the other and at a different figure. Check with your accountant and/or attorney for the best way to structure your business.)

This means that at some point in time, it may be advisable to restructure the business to take advantage of the tax breaks for that particular structure. Years ago, it was automatically assumed that forming a corporation was the only way to go. That is not the case any longer. Sometimes it is, sometimes it isn't, chiefly because of the tax codes that are always changing, depending on the political whim of the moment. Be aware and cognizant of the prevailing laws and codes so that when you achieve a different economic position, you are prepared to change the structure to take advantage. Again, this means working closely with your accountant.

Once again, let us bring up computers as a very useful tool in making future predictions and projections. Anything the computer program can achieve can also be done in longhand, only it takes much longer. Many planning functions can be performed in lightning speed with a few simple keystrokes that would take hours with pencil and paper.

A good spreadsheet program, for instance, can show you in seconds what the effect on net income would be by changing a single figure—increasing revenue by 12 percent or taxes by 8 percent—for the current year or a number of ensuing years. Another spreadsheet can show the depreciation schedules for hundreds of pieces of equipment. It can then print out various graphs that can help you decide what the best move would be, regarding every aspect of your business. As a forecasting tool, computers are unparalleled.

Suppose you wish to compare the effects of depreciation on profits and taxes using the sum-of-the-years-digits method versus the straight-line method, two common methods used. By changing a few figures you could have the result immediately, on the screen or printed out in a chart or graph. For an excellent description of personal computers and how they can be used in business, a very good text is *Your Small Business Made Simple*, Gallagher, Doubleday, 1989.

SETTING AND MEETING LONG-RANGE GOALS

At the end of each business year, you need to sit down with various people and critique the past year's performance and project goals for the coming year. Those goals should be compatible with longer-range goals, which should be reevaluated as well.

The first person to consult is your accountant. You will want to review your mission statement to be certain you are on track with your stated goals and philosophy. Then, you need to review your business plan and develop the plan for the coming year. You should develop an annual budget to aid you in achieving the profit levels you have set as your goal.

When you are satisfied with the direction you mean to take and have a plan in place to achieve the stated goals, then it is time to sit down with your staff and explain where the salon is and where it is headed, how they are included, what you expect from them, and what they can expect from you. Solicit input from them as well, as they may see ways of achieving your goals easier than you have. Including them in this process is also the most effective way of ensuring that they will work hard to achieve those goals, especially if they can be made to see that your goals will also be of benefit to them.

Learn to spot trends and capitalize on them. Major national and global trends are important to the salon business, and those that recognize and take advantage of them will profit the most. Books such as *Megatrends* by John Naisbitt, and *The Age Wave* by Ken Dychtwald, Ph.D., are highly recommended for predicting coming trends.

Examples of trends that will affect the salon business are:

- The over sixty-five age group is expanding rapidly while other age groups are decreasing.
- U.S. population is shifting to the South and the West.
- Baby boomers who have dominated every market since they came on the scene are now entering their fifth decade.
- Women are in the work force at all-time high levels.
- As the baby boomers enter middle age in more and more numbers, the industries associated with aging are projected to increase for the next half-century. We already see a significant rise in skin-care lines in our own industry, and there is an explosion in such fields as fitness, health, and nutrition, all of which we can capitalize upon.
- Couples are delaying having children, and 25 percent of all couples will elect not to have offspring.
- More than half of all humankind's information has been gained in the last fifty years. Technology is reshaping the world and creating more jobs than any other sector. Computers in the salon are here to stay, and it is going to be increasingly difficult to survive without such a system.

Monitor trade magazines for their predictions. They spend a great deal of time, money, and research to provide accurate forecasts for you. Their experience is invaluable and is provided for the mere cost of the magazine. Trade books, such as this one, are invaluable as well. Read, study, watch, and learn as much as you can about the changing world and our (hair salons') place in it.

REVIEW

When you find you can't keep up with demand, it is time to consider growing, which might mean offering expanded services. The more diversified you are, the less affected by sudden trends you'll be.

Another way to expand is to franchise your operation. Ensure that you are ready to expand when the time is right by providing for cash when you need it. Establish a positive credit rating. Tax planning can help provide you with necessary funds for further expansion, as well as demonstrate that you have control of your business. Review your goals at least annually, keeping trends in mind when you make your plans.

C H A P T E R
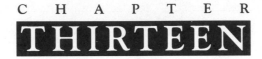
THIRTEEN

As we engage in what is primarily a service business, we are labor intensive and, as such, are limited by what we can produce within a finite amount of time. Only so many hours in a day, week, month, or year are available to us to be productive in, and, as we are not machines, after a given point we begin to exhaust ourselves and production levels fall. It makes sense then to use those business hours available to us to their best possible utilization. Intelligent time management is the key.

A quick look at the excellent reference publication, *Books In Print*, available in virtually all public libraries, will tell you that there are over sixty books on the single subject of time management still in print and still being sold. That many books on a relatively narrow topic tells us that this is indeed a serious subject and one worthy of your attention and study. A visit to the business reference section of your library will reveal dozens of books, pamphlets, and audio-visual materials on this subject, and the librarian will confirm that these sources are some of the most widely used. A look at the list of those checking out time management sources will probably reveal the names of individuals known to be good business people in your community.

You absolutely must manage your time efficiently if you have a desire to accomplish such things as:

- Make a lot of money.
- Spend a lot of time with your family.
- Get enough vacation and "off" time.
- Live to a ripe old age.

When you hear someone make a statement like, "Oh, my business doesn't allow me to spend a lot of time with my kids, but the time I do spend is quality time," they are buying into a myth a lot of people have bought into, and for the most part it is just that — a myth. If the time you are spending with your family is short, just because you pack a lot of action or activity into it doesn't make that time any higher quality than any other particular time, and many times is merely a way to excuse those uncomfortable guilt feelings that not being available as a parent or spouse can generate. (Figure 13.1)

When you first open your own business, you must expect to put in a tremendous amount of hours for at least the first year or so and perhaps longer. And being a salon owner will almost always mean that

FIGURE 13.1
Family time—one of the most important things effective management can bring you.

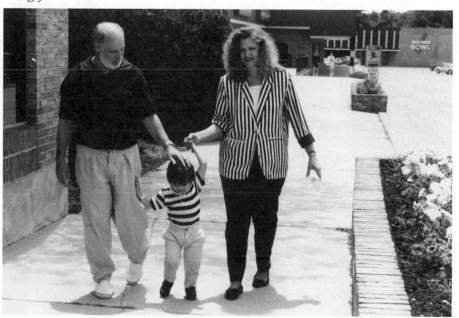

you will have to contribute more time to the business than your employees. But there should come a point when the business is staffed sufficiently so you can begin to devote plenty of time to your family and yourself and not to the business. If you have had your salon doors open for three to five years and you are still putting in eighty-hour weeks, then it is time (past time!) to begin learning some time management strategies. Let us hope that you are not in that state at present, but if you are, there are relatively easy ways to change the situation.

Think about this: If you find yourself saying to acquaintances, perhaps with a laugh, that you are "married to your business"—and you see more than a germ of truth to it—you may well find that your family eventually will not allow you to practice what has become a form of bigamy and will take measures to see that in the future you are wedded to only one of the parties.

The whole point is, one of the chief reasons most of us decide to open a salon is to eventually obtain a higher quality of life, and for the majority of us at least a partial definition of that goal would be to spend more time with our loved ones. Time management is the process by which we are able to spend the resource of time as we wish to spend it, *not* as a dictatorial business might demand.

When you run a one-person operation, it follows that you will have to do it all—perform the services that bring in the income and manage the business so that you have clients on whom to perform those services. Even then, labor- and time-saving devices and methods can make your job that much easier and afford you time for other pursuits and activities.

I mention computers throughout this book, chiefly because computers are not the wave of the future any longer; they are the wave of the present. Their chief attribute is that they can be used to save you time—time better spent to improve your salon, and time spent away from the salon!

A word of caution about computers, however. It is very tempting to let the computer become time-consuming in itself. For instance, computerizing your salon may save you enormous blocks of time in preparing taxes and payroll, inventory control, and all the other chores computers can do for us. If you are not careful, however, you can get swept up in the magic of the thing until you are spending all of your time playing with it, and the computer becomes counter-productive. You are no longer using it for what you intended—to simplify and ease your workload. You can become computer-obsessed and begin to neglect not only your family but perhaps your business as well by spending hours and hours on the humming gray box. Be aware of this danger and always remember a computer is merely a tool, even if it is a particularly fascinating one.

First of all, if you don't already know how, learn to do several things at once. I had a friend in the salon business who constantly complained of not having time for anything but his business. He was ready to sell what was a very profitable operation, because it was quite simply killing him. I visited him for a lunch date to talk over a joint business venture, and while I was waiting for him, I followed him around as he completed some last minute chores he wanted to do before we left. This is what he did. He walked into his shampoo area and rinsed out some perm rods that he had left in a sink. He dried them in a towel and then took them back to the area where they were stored. Then he went back out to the waiting area, picked up a dirty ashtray, took it back to the break room where he hunted up a soiled towel, cleaned it, and took it back out to the waiting area. His next move was to go over to his cutting area, clean out the dirty towels in the container, take them back to the laundry room, and deposit them in the washing machine. There wasn't enough for a full load, so he went back out to the cutting room and picked up an armful of dirty linen from another stylist's container, took them back, added them to the load, and then started the machine. By this time I was crazy!

"Sam," I said (not his name), "I see one reason right now why you never get out of here until midnight. You can't chew gum and walk at the same time." I smiled as I said it, but I was dead serious. I had known him for years and realized that this was the way he had always done things. What had taken him three or four different trips should have taken one or two at the most. He could have rinsed the rods, grabbed the ashtray in one hand on the way back, deposited the rods in their bin, cleaned the ashtray with the towel he'd just used, gotten all the dirty towels from everyone's bin in the cutting room, taken them back to the laundry room, made a load from them, and done everything it took three trips to accomplish in one. Learn to do several tasks at once, if you don't do that already. Life's too short to spend it making every little job a major production.

Listen to yourself when you make appointments. Do you spend five minutes finding a time for that client, perhaps naming every single time slot you have open, or do you guide him or her to the time you want to fill, quickly and easily?

Learn to use your time efficiently. Learn to prioritize. If you have a mental (or written) list of things you feel you have to do by eleven o'clock, don't allow that list to become the Ten Commandments. If something comes up that is more important, you need to update your priorities.

Here's an example. You are attending a seminar in two weeks in Chicago and during a lull in the morning's action pick up the phone to make your hotel reservations. The desk clerk puts you on hold and just then two people walk in the salon and start looking at the merchandise on the shelves. You had just spent ten minutes trying to get through to the hotel and it had been busy each time. Here is an opportunity to prioritize. Hang up the darned phone and take care of the clients! Sometime during the next week or so, chances are probably pretty good you'll get another lull and you can call the hotel back.

Let's say you don't do this. The clerk takes another five minutes to get back to you, and by then one client has left because no one has waited on him or her. The other has waited on him or herself and is standing before you waiting to pay, but you have to hold up your little pinkie and ask the customer to wait while you attempt to make a reservation with the clerk who's come back on and appears to have an IQ in the low two-digit range. Guess how many people are going to be upset and who has just lost at least one sale and the goodwill of probably both clients? Not to mention that by the time you finally make the reservation and ring up the sale, your next client has waited six minutes while watching you chat away on the phone. Prioritize!

Many books can teach you excellent time management skills, and you should read as many of them as you can. (See Appendix B for a partial list.) And keep reading these types of books as soon as they come out, as new and better techniques are constantly being discovered. If you read no other texts, be sure and read the *One Minute Manager* series of books by Kenneth Blanchard. They are excellent!

HOW EMPLOYEES AFFECT YOUR TIME

Once you have begun to hire employees, your work theoretically *should* begin to ease up, but many have found that the opposite is true. That is because they have not learned to use effective time management methods. Instead of having more time once new employees are added, the opposite seems to happen. The employees themselves begin to demand attention for their problems and the salon owner is forced to borrow time from his or her personal life. A forty- or fifty-hour workweek has just become a seventy- or eighty-hour stint. As Professor Harold Hill said in *The Music Man*, "there's trouble in River City, folks!"

This problem is relatively easy to diagnose, and the cure is proper time management. The owner or manager has less time than before, even though supposedly there are more hands to do the work, because he or she has made the mistake of shifting to his or her lap the problems that belong to the staff. This is a common malady but, unlike the common cold, there is a cure. The manager affected has to transfer the load back to its proper owner. That's not as difficult as it sounds. (Figure 13.2)

Here's an example of how employees create unnecessary work for the owner or manager: Betsy, the salon coordinator (receptionist par

FIGURE 13.2
Owners or managers who have accepted staffers' problems need to begin the time management technique of transferring the loads back to their rightful owners. That's not as difficult as it sounds.

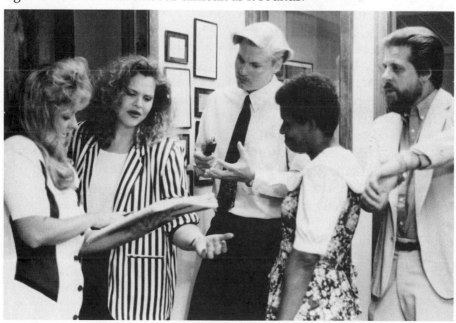

excellence!) comes back to where the owner, Nancy, is cutting a client's hair, and interrupts her with the "urgent" message, "Nancy, I just noticed that Acme Beauty Supply has been charging us sales tax on the products we purchase for resale. They're not supposed to do that, are they? What should we do about it?"

Nancy excuses herself to her customer, turns to Betsy, and says, "Why, gee, Betts, you're right, those dogs aren't supposed to do that! That's costing us a fortune! I'll take care of it as soon as I can. Thanks for letting me know."

There are several things wrong with this scenario, and I hope you picked them all out. If you did, skip ahead, for this is not your problem—you already know how to prevent employees from unloading problems that are their purview onto your shoulders. If, however, this sounds frighteningly familiar, read on.

First of all, the receptionist should not have chosen the time she did to inform her boss of the problem. This was not an urgent problem at all. It was one that needed addressing, but a few more hours or even another day or two would have meant very little. The receptionist needs to know that this sort of problem has a lower priority, certainly lower than the proper servicing of Nancy's client.

Second, this was not the owner's problem. This sort of crisis could certainly fall within Betsy's authority, depending on the salon and the owner's policy. If the position is that of a salon coordinator and not simply a receptionist, it certainly falls within her job description. Even so, it is perhaps legitimate for Betsy to at least inform Nancy of the problem, but Nancy took the wrong tack by accepting the problem, and as a result, accepted the responsibility for taking care of it, even though it shouldn't have been hers to begin with.

What she could, and should, have done was say to Betsy, "Betsy, you're right, that's not correct procedure, but this is not the time to talk about it. Remind me again of this when I have a free moment. Please don't forget." She then should have returned to her client.

Later, when Betsy reminded her of the problem at a more appropriate moment, she should have reinforced the lesson already given, by saying, "Betsy, I appreciate your coming to me with this problem, but you should have waited until I wasn't with a client to do so. This is a problem, but not an urgent one. Do you see that? Okay. Now, what do you suggest be done about it?"

At this point, Betsy, being an intelligent and thoughtful employee (after all, she did spot the problem, didn't she?) will probably come up with the right solution, which in this case would be to contact Acme, let them know of the problem, and determine what they are going to do about it. If their response is satisfactory, all that remains to be done is for Betsy to monitor their action to be sure they have rectified the situation and reimbursed the salon for any wrongful sales tax charges. By handling the situation in this manner, Nancy has handed the problem back to its rightful owner, who is perfectly capable of handling it, and is, in fact, being paid to perform this very kind of duty, and she has helped that employee grow, which will make her even more valuable. She has also eliminated the need to sacrifice some of her personal time to remedy the problem.

That is how time management works, at least one aspect of it. You not only have to learn to delegate authority, you have to learn who has what job and then give them the freedom and authority to do it. If you end up doing everyone else's job, then they are not given the opportunity and room to grow as employees, and you will increasingly have to use your own time to do their jobs as well as your own.

Here is a problem we recently had in our own salon that is an excellent example of taking on another person's load. A product line representative was visiting the salon and I took the opportunity to solicit his opinion on a better way to display his rack of merchandise. Picking up a bottle of shampoo to see how it would look in another location, I was dismayed to see a film of dust around it. Part of the co-designer's job in our salon is to dust each and every product bottle once weekly, an onerous chore as we carry over twenty product lines including our own, but a necessary duty and one we insist on.

I went to Janice, the senior co-designer, with my complaint, and I wasn't in a very happy state when I approached her. To my chagrin, she explained everything had been dusted according to schedule on Tuesday. As this was only Friday, I was skeptical of her defense, but soon learned that she was telling the truth. I felt badly about accusing her of not doing her job, especially as Janice happens to be one of the quickest learners I have ever had the pleasure to employ as well as being a very talented hairstylist who will be promoted to designer status faster than anyone ever has at our salon. She informed me that dust was a big problem, and frustrating since it seemed that no sooner had she finished cleaning than it was almost as if it had never been done, as the dust accumulated so quickly. She suspected the problem was a heating/air conditioning duct that needed its filter cleaned or replaced.

"Well," I said, after apologizing for unjustly accusing her of not performing her duties properly, "I'll call someone and get it checked out." A few minutes later it dawned on me that I had accepted a job that should have been hers. I called Janice back and asked her what she thought should be done. She suggested a filter service might be contacted to look at the ducts and that maybe one of them did that as a free service. "Good," I told her. "That's your project. Please take care of it."

She immediately phoned a company that sent someone out and gave a free estimate on cleaning the ducts and providing a filter service, and the problem was solved. Taking this project on and completing it gave her a heightened sense of accomplishment, she told me later, and it certainly was helpful to me because if she hadn't made the phone calls, talked to the estimator, and set up the contract to have the ducts cleaned, it would have fallen to me to do so, and we might still have dirty ducts and dusty product bottles. The problem was solved, an employee gained a measure of self-satisfaction in taking responsibility for a project, thereby raising her value as an employee, and I was able to go home on time, rather than remain behind for an hour after my last client to call duct-cleaning companies.

When employees are consistently leaving work earlier than the boss, then the boss needs to have a long, hard look at the method by which he or she manages time. Employees should *ease* the workload, not add to it. In fact, once a staff is in place, the owner should be the one going home early and the employees the ones putting in the long hours. Those extra hours many of us put in as owners are quite often spent not in doing *our* work, but our employees'. Employees aren't working for the owner; he or she is working for them! Not only that—when he or she finally gets home, family members are dumping their loads in his or her lap as well. Little Janey announces she has just been named one of the varsity cheerleaders and, upon congratulation, informs Mom she will need a ride to practice every Wednesday evening. Mom (salon owner) is such a nice person, she tells Janey she'll get on it right away and call some of the other parents to arrange a car pooling schedule.

This is a person with a real problem! She is doing everyone else's work at the salon, then she goes home and does her children's work as well. It never entered her head that perhaps little Janey could take the responsibility for arranging her own transportation. Do you see how it becomes an entire lifestyle?

The way out is simple. Let others do their own work. Don't take on other people's jobs. You have enough to do in performing your own. If you're afraid a change in your work philosophy may anger or irritate employees or family members, you may be right—after all, they've just lost their best employee—but then, you may be pleasantly surprised to learn that they are happy to take responsibility for their own jobs. By always doing the other person's job you are, in effect, saying to that person that you don't feel he or she is capable of doing it. By rescuing employees and even family members constantly, you actually end up preventing them from realizing their potential.

When you begin to utilize the resources you already have in the salon, your employees, you will begin to see them as solutions to problems, not the source of problems.

If you are guilty of doing everyone else's job, here's what you can do about it. First thing Tuesday morning (or Monday morning, or whatever morning is the first workday of the week), call your staff into your office or a private area, one by one, and apologize to them for taking over their jobs. Let them know that you will no longer do so and that you will from now on allow them to do their own jobs and allow them even more responsibility. You are going to be surprised. Most people welcome responsibility and work. Most of your employees are going to welcome your news. The ones who don't, if there are any, well . . . to heck with them. After all, you're the boss, aren't you?

Years ago I took a break from the hair business for a year and worked as a headhunter (recruiter) for the high-voltage recruiting firm of Kendall & Davis, Inc. This company was and is recognized as one of the top companies of its kind in the nation. When I worked there, it had two sides; one part of the company recruited electronics engineers (E.E.s) strictly within the field of electronic warfare and within the entire country, and the other side recruited data processing people within a contiguous five-state area. One of the unique things about the company's recruiting philosophy, and the source of its strength, was that it took a different tack than corporate personnel departments. At that time, most companies' hiring procedures were to call down to personnel and announce a job, and the personnel people would then request a job description. From the job description, they would identify, say, ten tasks the person to fill the job would have to do. They would then attempt to locate a qualified person by various means—posting within the company, blind ads, a search through files for resumes, etc.

Kendall & Davis, on the other hand, took a different view. If the job called for a person to be able to perform ten tasks, it didn't look for a person capable of doing all ten. Instead it searched for someone who could do six or seven of the ten and was capable of learning how to do the remaining tasks. For the prospective employee, the job then became much more attractive as it was now a career-enhancing opportunity, rather than a lateral job switch. This accomplished several very positive things. First, it was a much more interesting job for the new hire as he or she would be learning new skills, thereby making him or herself a more valuable professional with the acquisition of the newly learned skills. That also made for a much happier employee, as he or she felt very useful and needed. When people grow in a job, it makes all the difference in the world in their attitude.

Second, it was great for the company making the hire. It got a person with growth potential and a positive attitude. When employees make a job change that is in essence a parallel move, they usually are moving for the basest of all reasons—more money. That is probably the worst reason of all to change jobs. Most times all a company gets in such employees (with that sole motive in hiring on) are malcontents, and chances are good to excellent they will move on again the first time another company waves the money carrot under their noses.

Take a page from Kendall & Davis. It isn't one of the most successful recruiting firms in the country by accident. Make sure the people you hire fit the same philosophy. Employees you hire that change to your salon from another solely because they see your salon as their avenue to more money may not be the right kind of people to add to your staff. On the other hand, persons that see it as a place to make more money because they will be given an opportunity to increase their knowledge and abilities—those kinds of people you should grab!

After you meet with your people, advising them of your new policy, then follow up by giving them expanded duties. Let the salon coordinator or receptionist do the daily books and basic accounting tasks. Once he or she is capable of performing those extra duties, he or she is no longer just a receptionist, but now can list "simple bookkeeping" among his or her job skills.

Give that stylist with a flair for expression the chance to work up some copy for your new ad campaign. Give that stylist the ball and let him or her run with it. It will take another chore from you and expand that person's skills so that when opening his or her own salon the stylist will know how to write an effective ad. If the stylist has skills in that area but doesn't have a clue how to write ad copy, suggest he or she go to the library, research the topic, and then come up with a good ad in seven days. You will be surprised at the alacrity the staff member may exhibit in rushing off to perform the task.

These are just suggestions to give you ideas. Everyone on your staff has skills and abilities you should be tapping, both for your benefit and for theirs. Take pains to show them how this will enhance them as well and solicit their input as to how else you can use them. You may well have a closet bean-counter among your people who would like nothing better than to run your inventory control system, or a budding Erte who can turn out better artwork for your yellow pages ad than the drudge down at the advertising agency. Put your people to work with not only their obvious hairstyling skills, but other talents as well.

In your training program, are you using senior stylists to conduct training sessions, or are you still doing that yourself? Go home, put your feet up, toss the baby in the air, knowing that your training is in good hands. After all, didn't you train your senior people yourself?

When you stop by to chat with your staff and they don't have time to talk as they are busy handling clientele and other job-related chores, then you are managing your time effectively.

Don't simply give staff members jobs and forget it. Follow up by creating a deadline for completion of the project and give them whatever authority is needed to fully accomplish the job. If you give someone the responsibility for creating an ad, review the ad when completed, and take some action. Either request it be improved if it doesn't fit the parameters or standards you set up, or if it fits the bill, use it. Run the ad. What greater source of pride for that employee, and what greater way to reward him or her than by using the fruit of his or her labor!

Your job as a salon owner is not to bring in all the salon's income, but to manage it. Jobs such as bookkeeping, accounting, inventory tracking and control, and so on are essential, vital, and necessary, but are basically routine tasks that ought not be the purview of the manager. Those functions should be delegated to others so that you can better direct the company, which is what a manager ought to be doing. Granted, keeping the books is very important—just ask the IRS!—but you don't think General Motors asks the president of the company to perform that task, no matter how necessary, do you? Of course not—his or her job is to steer the company and make decisions that will affect its future. When you first begin the business, naturally you will have to do all of the jobs involved in the running of a small business, but as you add staff, those functionary chores should be given to others so that you may devote your more valuable time to making the salon grow.

This is a lesson many never learn. How many salon owners do you know who constantly excuse themselves from their clients to talk to salespeople, distributors, clients, and others, and then spend long hours at night entering the daily totals in their ledgers? More than there should be. Perhaps this is one of the reasons many of us burn out or have salons that never seem to grow past a certain point. Give those onerous chores up! Remember, the only way to develop responsibility in people is to give it to them.

It becomes obvious that to manage effectively you must have quality personnel on board. Making sure you get those people initially is half the battle, but we all make mistakes in hiring. An interview situation is essentially a "romance" situation, in which both sides are pitching woo to the other, and as such, is perhaps not a good method to judge how a prospective employee will work out. Be very careful with your hires.

DEVELOPING YOUR STAFF

Once you have staff, you need to be aware of both the contributors and those bodies merely occupying space. The deadwood, in other words. Such employees will do nothing but drag the entire salon down, and will become the chief source of your problems, thereby stealing time away from your outside life.

For instance, you may have two stylists, both fully booked, both having been on board a significant period of time, say, two years. If one employee is doing a great deal of walk-ins and/or clients that were initially referred by other stylists in the salon, while the other employee's clientele is composed of referrals he or she has hustled from other clients, then it doesn't require a genius to figure out which employee is contributing and which isn't. It is safe to bet that the one who is simply servicing clients given to him or her is also going to be the source of most of your problems. You have three choices with such an employee. You can simply ignore the situation. You can attempt to help him or her change the situation, which may lead to the third choice if he or she cannot or will not turn the situation around, which is to terminate the employee. If all a staffer is doing is servicing clientele already there and not adding clientele from this source, then he or she is a body occupying space and is holding the salon back from increasing its potential. You have a hard decision to make. You can be either a "good guy" or a good business person. Firing someone should always be a last resort. You should make every effort and attempt you possibly can to resolve the situation, but if it comes to it, a good manager sometimes has to make difficult decisions, unless the growth and health of the business are not important concerns.

The point is, many of us who are salon owners need to begin to do some managing, instead of being managed. We must remember there is another part of that very true saying, "Time is money." Time is also *life*, and when your time runs out . . . that's it, pal.

Manage your time to its best and most satisfying use.

Some famous comments on time:

"Time is just the space between our memories. When we cease perceiving this space, time has vanished." Henri Frederic Amiel in *Diary,* January 21, 1866.

"Time is the sole capital of people whose only fortune is their intelligence." Honore de Balzac.

"One can forget time only by making use of it." Baudelaire, *My Heart Laid Bare.*

"Time is invention or it is nothing at all." Henri Bergson, French philosopher.

"Thus, time makes me and I make time." Marie Antoinette, sometime prior to her beheading (I assume).

(My personal favorite) "Time is the substance I am made of. Time is a river that sweeps me along, but I am time; it is a tiger that rips me apart, but I am the tiger; it is a fire that consumes me, but I am the fire." Jorge Luis Borges in *Other Inquisitions.*

"It is not time that is lacking, it is we who are lacking it." Paul Claudel in *Partage de midi.*

"Because I know that time is always time
And place is always and only place
And what is actual is actual only for one time
And only for one place
I rejoice that things are as they are." T.S. Eliot in *Ash Wednesday*.

"We have forgotten that our only goal is to live and that we live each day and that at every hour of the day we are reaching our true goal if we are living . . . The days are fruits and our role is to eat them." Jean Giono in *Fullness of Days*.

"The standardization of time is the basis of a classificatory system that rules life. Except for birth and death, all important activities are scheduled." E. Hall in *Beyond Culture*.

Here's one definitely for the salon owner

"In fact, being in a position to decide the use of one's time—and the hours one is present at the office—indicates that one has arrived." Ibid.

"Because nothing is more precious than time, there is no greater generosity than to lose it without counting." Marcel Jouhandeau in *Everyday Occurrences*.

"Time is a sort of river of passing events, and strong is its current." Marcus Aurelius Antoninus, Roman emperor, in *Meditations IV.*

"It is possible that for persons who use their time well, knowledge and experience increase throughout life." Michel de Montaigne in *Essays, Book I.*

"Time is the great art of man." Napoleon Bonaparte in *Letters to the King of Naples*.

"We don't want to miss anything in our time; perhaps there are finer times, but the present one is ours." Jean Paul Sartre in *Situations II.*

"We ought always to see ourselves as people who are going to die the next day. It is the time we think we have before us that kills." Elsa Triolet in *Luna Park*.

"Time is long enough to whoever takes advantage of it; He who works and thinks stretches its limits." Voltaire in *Discourse in Verse on Man*.

"Time is the most beautiful thing with its ruins, its thromboses, its vanished hopes, its illusions that die, and gives each breaking day a new illusion . . ." Ettore Scola.

It becomes evident that a lot of intelligent people have recognized the value of time and the management of it.

REVIEW

Time management is necessary if you want to make a lot of money, spend time with your family, have time off of work, and live a long life. When you first open a salon, you can expect to put in long hours, but this shouldn't continue for years. Learn to use time efficiently, and learn to prioritize.

Once you hire employees, your work should begin to ease up, as long as you don't make your employees' problems your own. Develop responsibility in your employees by giving them responsibilities.

APPENDIX A

Creating a salon from scratch can begin to seem like an impossibly daunting task at times, especially to someone who has never before attempted such an ambitious undertaking. Granted, there are dozens of ingredients—some complex and some relatively simple—that are necessary before a successful business can be launched, but fortunately there is plenty of help available out there for the uninitiated. Don't despair!

SCORE AND ACE

Two of the top organizations for aiding start-up small businesses are the Service Corps of Retired Executives (SCORE) and the Active Corps of Executives (ACE). Both groups are independent, national, nonprofit organizations of retired and active business people who volunteer their time to provide free counseling and low-cost training to prospective entrepreneurs and small business owners.

SCORE is sponsored by the Small Business Administration (SBA), and their primary purpose is to assist those who are thinking about or have recently started their own business. Their counseling activities generally do not include technical assistance, but place their emphasis on the specific management skills and business planning necessary in starting and running a business. The counselors in SCORE come from a variety of business and industry backgrounds and a specific SCORE volunteer who has experience in a relevant or start-up business may work with the new business owner for an extended period of time if needed. This counseling is worth its weight in gold, especially to a neophyte business owner. Your local SCORE affiliate can be located by perusing the phone book or by contacting the Small Business Administration office in your area.

ACE counselors as a rule are not involved in counseling sessions but serve as guest speakers at SCORE workshops, providing expert advice. These professionals are active business professionals from the community and are usually very successful in their businesses and therefore have good tips and advice to pass on.

CHAMBERS OF COMMERCE

Your local chambers of commerce are another valuable source of aid, information, and business expertise. Their mission is to support existing businesses, better the civic and economic vitality of the community through public education programs, and promote the growth and development of commercial, industrial, and professional enterprises. Chambers are typically independent, voluntary associations of business persons and are funded by membership dues and fees rather than tax monies. They are not affiliated with local government or accountable to any other organizations.

Chambers of commerce work with other organizations for community betterment and enhancement of goodwill among citizen, government, education, and business groups, also offering support for women, minorities, and small business owners.

Membership in your local chamber is usually a wise investment, giving you access to referral services; networking opportunities; business and membership directory; free notary service; research service that provides excellent demographic and statistical information; community materials in the form of maps, brochures, and fact sheets; business seminars; and many other services.

You can locate your local chamber in the phone book or by contacting the state chamber of commerce in your state's capital.

LIBRARIES

Your local library is an abundant source of information and aid for businesses. If you live in a sizeable community, your library will probably contain a separate section or division on business or business and technology that will be loaded with valuable information on business in general and your type of business in particular. Even if a particular title may not be on hand at your branch, it can usually be obtained through a number of methods such as interlibrary loans. If you are unfamiliar with research methods, talk to the librarian or resource person. These professionals are among the friendliest and most helpful in the universe, in my experience! Don't be afraid that your request or question might be a dumb one and neglect to ask it. Best of all—libraries represent a *free* resource! (Figure A.1)

SMALL BUSINESS DEVELOPMENT CENTERS (SBDC)

Each state has a statewide business assistance service offering one-on-one counseling at no cost and other assistance through training

FIGURE A.1
Use your local library. It's a great resource!

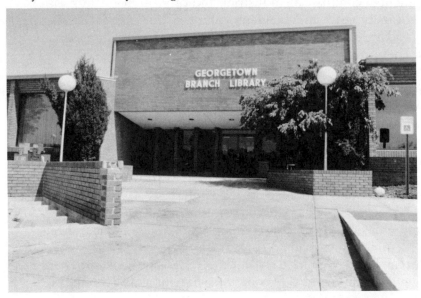

programs and seminars to small business owners. Planning and problem solving are just two of the areas in which SBDCs can help. Call the state office of the chamber of commerce if an SBDC is not listed in your local phone book.

THE SMALL BUSINESS ADMINISTRATION (SBA)

The SBA is an independent federal agency Congress set up in 1953, and its basic role is to assist, counsel, and champion the millions of American small businesses that are the backbone of this country's competitive free enterprise economy. Everybody likes to talk about the Fortune 500 type of companies because they are so huge, glamorous, and visible, but the truth is, small business accounts for the lion's share of American business and the economy.

A chief role of the SBA is in offering a variety of programs to eligible small business concerns that cannot borrow on reasonable terms from conventional lenders such as banks and credit unions without government help. SBA's primary mission is to help people get into and stay in business. To this end, the SBA acts as an advocate for small business, explains small business' role and contributions to our society and economy, and advocates programs and policies that will aid and succor small business. To perform this role, the SBA works in close cooperation with other federal agencies and Congress, and with educational, financial, professional, and trade institutions and organizations.

Most SBA business loans are made by private banks and lenders and are guaranteed by the agency. Most small, independent businesses are eligible for SBA assistance, as are homeowners, renters, and nonprofit organizations. The SBA makes special efforts to assist minorities, women, and veterans to start up and stay in business since such persons have traditionally faced unusual difficulties in the private sector.

The SBA provides free and low-cost publications to assist small business persons in their business planning. Topics include financial management and analysis, general management and planning, and marketing. In October 1982, the SBA set up the Small Business Answer Desk to help callers with questions on how to start and manage a business, where to get financing, and other pertinent information needed to start and manage a business and to operate and expand a business. The toll-free number is (800) 827-5722.

To purchase an SBA publication send a check or money order (no cash, credit cards, or purchase orders) payable to the Small Business Administration, SBA Publications, P.O. Box 30, Denver, CO 80201-0030. Indicate the publications you want and include your name and mailing address.

Following is a partial list of the publications available:

Financial Management and Analysis

1. FM 1 *ABC's of Borrowing.* $1.00. The fundamentals of borrowing.
2. FM 3 *Basic Budgets for Profit Planning.* $.50. Budgeting system.
3. FM 4 *Understanding Cash Flow.* $1.00. Plan for cash requirements.
4. FM 5 *Venture Capital Primer.* $.50. Venture capital resources.
5. FM 7 *Analyze Your Records to Reduce Costs.* $.50. Add efficiency.
6. FM 8 *Budgeting in a Small Service Firm.* $.50. Keep financial records.
7. FM 9 *Sound Cash Management and Borrowing.* $.50. Cash management.
8. FM 10 *Record Keeping in a Small Business.* $1.00. Record keeping.
9. FM 11 *Break-Even Analysis: A Decision Making Tool.* Make decisions for sales, profits, and costs.
10. FM 12 *A Pricing Checklist for Small Retailers.* $.50. Pricing strategies.
11. FM 13 *Pricing Your Products and Services Profitably.* $1.00. Use various pricing techniques.

General Management and Planning

1. MP 1 *Effective Business Communications.* $.50 The role of business communication.
2. MP 2 *Locating or Relocating Your Business.* $1.00. Location selection.
3. MP 3 *Problems in Managing a Family-Owned Business.* $.50. Overcoming potential problems.
4. MP 6 *Planning and Goal Setting for Small Business.* $.50. Plan success.
5. MP 9 *Business Plan for Retailers.* $1.00. Develop a business plan.
6. MP 10 *Choosing a Retail Location.* $1.00. Location selection.
7. MP 16 *How to Buy or Sell a Business.* $1.00. Business valuation.
8. MP 20 *Business Continuation Planning.* $1.00. Life insurance needs.

U.S. POSTAL SERVICE

The Postal Service provides mail and parcel delivery services that can benefit your business. For example, if you are planning bulk mailings of your newsletter or a flyer or coupon, check with its account representative for ways to save you money. The Post Office will also standardize your computer data base diskettes to include zip + 4 coding, carrier route identification, and address standardization. This service is a must for salons wanting to save postage and ensure fast and accurate delivery of materials.

APPENDIX B

Listed here are selected readings and other resource materials pertaining to the subject matter of this book that I have reviewed and believe to be of value. Many of the texts selected amplify in greater detail the subjects covered in this book, and should be of additional benefit to those wishing to explore a particular subject in more detail than can be provided in *Managing Your Business.*

The reviewed materials are listed by subject according to their primary topic, although some of the texts may have valuable information on other subjects as well. Many titles were researched, but only those thought to be of particular value to hairstylists are included. This is by no means an exhaustive listing as there is no way to be aware of every publication available, and more than likely many deserving titles have not been included. Apologies extended for any such omissions. New materials are published all the time, and it is suggested that salon entrepreneurs utilize their libraries, bookstores, and trade publications as a frequent source in the search for more knowledge.

> "Show me a man who has become a success, and
> I'll show you a man who had help getting there."
>
> C.L. Smith

ADVERTISING AND MARKETING

Books

- Baty, Gordon. *Entrepreneurship: Playing to Win.* Reston, Va.: Reston Publishing, 1974. The nuts and bolts of life in the small business lane.
- Day, William H. *Maximizing Small Business Profits.* Englewood Cliffs, N.J.: Prentice-Hall, 1978. Sound techniques to increase the bottom line.
- Dean, Sandra Linville. *How to Advertise: A Handbook for Small Businesses.* Wilmington, Del.: Enterprise Publishing, 1980. Good text for the basics.
- Kuswa, Webster. *Big Paybacks from Small-Budget Advertising.* Chicago: Dartnell, 1982. Nuggets of information.
- Levinson, Jay Conrad. *Guerrilla Marketing, Secrets for Making Big Profits from Your Small Business.* Boston: Houghton Mifflin Company, 1984. Absolutely the finest book of its kind on the market. A must read for the salon owner who is serious about marketing his or her business.
- Levinson, Jay Conrad. *Guerrilla Marketing Weapons.* New York: Plume Books-NAL-Dutton, 1990. One hundred ways to maximize profits—every time Levinson writes a book it's a hit!
- Malickson, David L., and John W. Nason. *Advertising—How to Write the Kind that Works.* New York: Charles Scribner's Sons, 1977. Fantastic tome to help you create the copy that will help sell your services.
- Ogilvy, David. *Ogilvy on Advertising.* New York: Crown Publishers, 1983. One of the "bibles" on the subject of advertising, large or small.
- Schollhammer, H., and Arthur Kuriloff. *Entrepreneurship and Small Business Management.* New York: John Wiley & Sons, 1979. Excellent reference.
- Siegel, Connie McClung. *How to Advertise and Promote Your Small Business.* New York: John Wiley & Sons, 1978. Good tips.
- Smith, Cynthia S. *How to Get Big Results from a Small Advertising Budget.* New York: Hawthorn Books, 1973. An older text but still applicable. Sound techniques never age—they just get painted a different color.
- Todd, Alden. *Finding Facts Fast: How to Find Out What You Want to Know Immediately.* Berkeley: Ten Speed Press, 1979. One of the

best texts for finding info quickly and painlessly. If you want to know how many permanent waves were sold last year, this book will tell you where to find that fact.

Periodicals

- *Advertising Age,* 740 N. Rush St., Chicago, IL 60611-2590. Read the pros and learn!
- *American Demographics,* P.O. Box 68, Ithaca, NY 14851. Great research on emerging buying trends and how to use the data for planning.
- *Barter Communique,* Full Circle Marketing Corp., P.O. Box 2527, Sarasota, FL 33578. Articles on how to barter for advertising on radio and television.
- *The Counselor Magazine,* Advertising Specialty Institute, NBS Bldg., 1120 Wheeler Way, Langhorne, PA 19047. Don't get a subscription, but you might want to peruse it at your library. Sometimes has good articles on specialty advertising.
- *More Business,* 11 Wimbledon Court, Jericho, NY 11753. Advertising articles of general interest—usually good ideas on incentive advertising and public relations material.
- *VM + SD (Visual Merchandising and Store Design),* ST Publications, 407 Gilbert Ave., Cincinnati, OH 45202. Great for product and merchandise presentation and advertising. Wonderful tips on how to display and present products that would cost thousands of dollars if you paid for these ideas. A great secret to be in on.

BOOKKEEPING

Books

- Fields, Louise W. Revised by Richard R. Gallagher. *Bookkeeping Made Simple.* New York: Doubleday, 1990. The best text I've found for understanding basic accounting, written in easy-to-understand language.
- Ragan, Robert, C.P.A. *Step-by-Step Bookkeeping, Rev. Ed., The Complete Handbook for the Small Businessman.* New York: Sterling Publishing, 1987. Good, basic text.

Software

- QuickBooks by Quicken. The best small business accounting software available, in my opinion. *PC Magazine* gives it its Editor's Award. This is a program that is extremely user-friendly and is also designed for the nonaccountant as no accounting knowledge is ever needed. You just fill out familiar looking checks, invoices, and check registers. Knowledge of double-entry accounting is not necessary, although the system will print out reports in that form for those who require it, such as banks. If you have a computer, this package may be the best purchase you make.

BUDGETING

Articles

- Beard, Larry H. "Economic Profit Maximization and Breakeven Analysis." *University of Michigan Business Review,* Vol. 29, Sept. 1977, pp. 18–22. Good treatise on how to reach your breakeven figures for products or services.
- Mesaros, Stanley J. "Expense Control Through Effective Budgeting." *Retail Control,* Vol. 46, June–July 1978, pp. 38–52. Good technical on eliminating waste from your product and service costs.
- Otley, David T. "Behavioral Considerations in Present Budgeting Systems." *Managerial Planning,* No. 49, Summer 1977. Scholarly presentation of how various factors influence costs.
- Smith, August W. "Effects of Variable Costing in Breakeven Analysis." *National Public Accountant,* Vol. 21, July 1976, pp. 12–14. Good article that explains variable costs when figuring breakeven points in cost analysis.

BUSINESS PLANS

Books

- Crego, Edwin T. Jr., Brian Deaton, and Peter D. Schiffrin. *How to Write a Business Plan, Second Edition.* Boston: American Management Association, 1986. One of the most comprehensive texts on the subject available. For the business planner who wants a truly sophisticated document, this is the book to consult.

- Delaney, Robert V. Jr. and Robert A. Howell. *How to Prepare an Effective Business Plan: A Step-by-Step Approach.* Boston: AMACOM, a division of American Management Association, 1986. A sound book, perhaps a bit advanced for our uses. Good for an in-depth understanding of a business plan, but more for manufacturing businesses than small service businesses.

Other Sources

Local libraries and local chapters of organizations such as SCORE and the Small Business Administration.

COMPUTERS

Books

- Gallagher, Richard R. *Your Small Business Made Simple.* New York: Doubleday, 1989. One of the best books you can get your hands on for learning all about personal computers (PCs) and how they can be used in your business.

Periodicals

- *PC Novice, Personal Computers in Plain English.* Subscriber Services—1(800)848-1478. PC Novice, P.O. Box 85380, Lincoln, NE 68501. This is the best darned magazine around for someone who knows little or nothing about computers. To quote from the magazine itself, "*PC Novice* is designed to give computer newcomers the basic information they need to begin using personal computers. We're a 'PC Primer,' an educational tool that teaches fundamentals. After someone knows the basics and is comfortable with their PC, they are ready to move up to the broader world of our sister publication *PC Today.* How will you know when you're ready to move up to *PC Today*? The items on the PC Novice Checklist (included in each issue) should help. Run down the list each month and check off the terms you don't recognize or understand. With each issue your list of unknown terms will get smaller and smaller. Also listed are general knowledge questions to test your knowledge. When you can recognize all the terms and answer the General Knowledge questions, you'll know you're ready to move up to *PC Today*, and may then switch your subscription to that magazine by phoning (800) 848-1478. There is no charge for this service." That pretty well says it all! An easy, inexpensive way to learn about computers. The articles are plainly written and easy to understand.

- *PC Magazine*, P.O. Box 54093, Boulder, CO 80322-4093. For subscription information, phone 1(800)289-0429 in the United States and Canada. $44.97 per year. Canada and other countries add $32.00 for postage. The standard of the industry, this is a very good publication for all PC user levels. One word of caution. *PC Magazine* judges and awards virtually everything there is in the computing world, and its award is a highly sought prize by manufacturers, distributors, wholesalers, mail order firms, computer outlets, and anyone else who stands to gain a buck by selling computer products. As it (*PC Magazine*) makes much of its income by selling ads to these same companies, it never really "bad-mouths" a product. The most you will see is a sort of "damning by faint praise." Rarely will it come right out and say a product is plain bad. Keep this in mind when reading product reviews and realize that the products placing lower may be worse than the magazine cares to say. This is not always true either, but would probably be a fairly good rule of thumb to apply when reading the reviews. Also, as the writers and editors are on the cutting edge of the industry, sometimes they have a lower opinion of products that have a bit of age on them. They will come out with editorials and articles that condemn perfectly valid products simply because, in the writers' opinions, they are now passe. This is a nice view if you always have access to the latest products and cost is no concern, but most of our budgets don't permit the purchase of everything new that comes down the pike, and our basic systems may have to last years, which is something they sometimes fail to take into account. This sounds like a blast at the publication, but please don't take it that way. This is probably the finest magazine of its kind in the marketplace, and except for the two points brought up here, an exemplary magazine with state-of-the-art information about the PC industry, and well worth the price of each copy.

- *Home Office Computing.* Scholastic, Inc., 730 Broadway, New York, NY 10003. Columns on sales, marketing, desktop publishing, business opportunities, resources, hardware/software reviews, other updates on computer use in the home and small businesses.
- Check local newsstands and bookstores for periodicals in the computer section. There are many general magazines as well as specialized magazines for the owners of particular hard- or software systems. Reading the ads in the computer magazines is a good learning experience, even for a novice. The more ads you read (and articles, of course!) the more you will begin to understand.

FINANCING

Books

- Alarid, William. *Money Sources for Small Business.* Santa Maria, Calif.: PUMA Publications, 1991. Decent reference to standard sources of financing for small businesses. No surprises here, but handy addresses for traditional sources as well as some basics for applying for funds. One nice thing about Alarid's book is that he lists sources by state.
- Blechman, Bruce, and Jay Conrad Levinson. *Guerrilla Financing, Alternative Techniques to Finance Any Small Business.* Boston: Houghton Mifflin Company, 1991. This could well be the most important book you'll ever check out of the library or buy! This is the nitty-gritty, down-to-earth bible on how to come up with the bucks to finance your salon. Reading this easy-to-understand-and-put-into-practice book will earn you a "Masters in Creative Financing" and dispel many of the myths most of us hold, such as "the only way you can get a bank loan is to prove you don't need it." This is as good a point as any to suggest you get your hands on any other of Jay Conrad Levinson's books—fourteen at last count, and all veritable fonts of small business wisdom.

Periodicals

- *New Business Opportunities.* Entrepreneur Group, Inc., 2392 Morse Ave., Irvine, CA 92714, (714) 261-2083. Monthly providing info on starting a small business and profiles of those who have done so successfully. How-to articles on starting up small businesses.

Other Sources

- *The Capital Institute.* The largest small-business financing firm in the hemisphere, founded by Bruce Jan Blechman, co-author of *Guerrilla Financing.* Besides arranging many different types of financing (for a fee, of course!), they offer other related services, such as financing consulting, financing and business plans, loan packaging, investor research reports, finding debt and equity sources of capital for your business, and slide and video presentations. For information, phone 1(800)748-6887.

FRANCHISES

Books

- Foster, Dennis L. *The Complete Franchise Book.* Rocklin, Calif.: Prima Publishers, 1987. A top-notch guide on how to assess a franchise and determine if a particular franchise is the best deal for your investment. Shows you what to look for—the pitfalls *and* the benefits of going the franchise route.

HOME-BASED SALONS

Periodicals

- *Homeworking Mothers.* Mothers' Home Business Network, Box 423, East Meadow, NY 11554, (516) 997-7394. Written for mothers who have home businesses and those who want to work at home so they can spend more time with their children. Advice and tips on taxes, marketing, and how to cope with working at home, among other topics.

LEASING

Companies and Other Sources

- Belvedere Company, One Belvedere Boulevard, Belvedere, IL 61008-8596, United States 1(800)435-5492; Canada 1(800)521-5147.
- Century Financial Services Group Ltd., 15455 Conway Road, Suite 350, Chesterfield, MO 63017.
- Local phone book (white and yellow pages) under Leasing.

MARRIAGE (AND OTHER ROOMMATES) AND RUNNING A BUSINESS TOGETHER.

Books

- Nelton, Sharon. *In Love and In Business.* New York: Wiley, 1986. How to run a business with your spouse—deadly serious and deadly humorous!

Periodicals

- *Home Sweet Home.* P.O. Box 1254, Milton, WA 98354. Fair quarterly that gives, among other gleanings, advice on interpersonal relationships in busy households. Worth an occasional read in your library.
- *Working Mother Magazine.* Lang Communications, 230 Park Ave., New York, NY 10169, (212) 551-9500. For the woman working outside the home who is trying to balance a career with the concerns of parenting. Usually at least one dramatic story each issue about a working mother that will make all who read it feel uplifted and inspired.

PERSONNEL

Books

- Middlemist, R. Dennis, and Michael A. Hitt. *Personnel Management: Jobs, People and Logic.* Englewood Cliffs, N.J.: Prentice-Hall, 1983. Understandable and helpful text.
- Moawad, Karen, and Michael Spence. *Personnel Manual for the Dental Office.* PennWell Books, 1985. Even though this is a dentist's book, the same principles apply to any service business. Lots of goodies here.
- Roxe, Linda A. *Personnel Management for the Smaller Company, A Hands-On Manual.* New York: AMACOM, 1979. Helpful reference guide.

SOFTWARE

- EmployeeManual*Maker,* by JIAN, Tools for Sales, 127 Second Street, Top Floor, Los Altos, CA 94022, (415) 941-9191. The perfect software program to develop a salon personnel manual;

a template in which you plug the specific information about your company and the policies you wish implemented. This program makes the whole process of compiling a personnel manual easy, effortless, and painless! Also, the writers of this program have taken special pains to create a document that is as friendly as possible toward the employee. Rather than a "Hey, you work here so toe the line or else . . . ," it is written with the attitude that says, "Hi! Welcome to our team. We've been here awhile and many things have been worked out . . . here's how we've agreed to manage our relationship . . ." A firm but friendly approach. Included are not only the Employee Manual template but chapters in the documentation book on finding good people, selecting good people, interview questions, application forms, new employee orientation, performance evaluation forms, and articles on wrongful termination, drug testing, family leave, sexual harassment, and the Americans with Disabilities Act. A great package for any salon no matter the size.

PLANNING

Books

- Davis, Stanley M. *Future Perfect.* Reading, Mass.: Addison-Wesley, 1987. As a business forecaster, Davis is among the best. See what the future holds for our industry and plan accordingly.
- *Any* book written by Peter F. Drucker, the forecaster who is always on the cutting edge in predicting future trends. Get whatever his latest book is.
- Grandt, Steven. *Entrepreneuring—The Ten Commandments for Building a Growth Company.* Reading, Mass.: Addison-Wesley, 1988. Blueprint that works.
- Sherman, James R. *Plan for Success.* Pathway Books. Excellent motivater and guide for the future.

Periodicals

- *Nation's Business.* Chamber of Commerce of the United States, 1615 H St. NW, Washington, D.C. 20062. Great magazine chock-full of useful information for small to medium business owners about managing their business.

Other Sources

- *CompuServe.* One of the computer services available for a monthly charge for basic services and additional charges for various other services. To avail yourself of CompuServe and other computer services, such as Prodigy, GEnie, and others, you must have a computer, modem, communications software, and a telephone. Among other handy and useful references, such as on-line computer forums, E-mail, news, weather, sports, the Associated Press wire, Business Wire, Consumer Reports, and so on, CompuServe offers a plethora of business services and assistance sources, such as International Entrepreneur's Network, Business Demographics, Business Database, U.S. Government Publications, Public Relations and Marketing, and Information USA. One of their most interesting and useful features offered is a vital planning tool called SUPERSITE Demographic Information. Simply type in the zip code of whatever area you are researching, and this service will provide a detailed and superior quality demographic report, for a per-report charge of from $10 to $100.

PUBLIC RELATIONS

Books

- Davidow, William, and Bro Uttal. *Total Customer Service, The Ultimate Weapon.* New York: Harper and Row, 1989. Great book to help you structure a winning philosophy toward your clientele.
- Louis, H. Gordon. *How to Handle Your Own Public Relations.* Chicago: Nelson Hall, 1976. Valuable and instructive.
- Rein, Irving, Phillip Kotler, and Martin Stoller. *High Visibility.* New York: Dodd, Mead, 1987. Readable and entertaining— tells methods of making your image better known.
- Sewell, Carl, and Paul Brown. *Customers for Life.* New York: Pocket Books, 1990. Exhilarating read on how to obtain and create loyal clients.

QUALITY CONTROL IN THE SALON

Books

- Bowles, Jerry, and Joshua Hammond. *Beyond Quality: How 50 Winning Companies Use Continuous Improvement.* New York: Putnam, 1991. Learn by example from the best.

SALES TECHNIQUES AND METHODS

Books

- Carew, Jack. *You'll Never Get No for an Answer.* New York: Simon & Schuster, 1987. Rich in positive thinking and how to get the client to buy.
- Delmar, Ken. *Winning Moves.* New York: Warner Books, 1984. Body language useful for selling.

SMALL BUSINESS IN GENERAL

Books

- *The MacMillan Small Business Handbook.* Various contributors— New York: MacMillan Press, 1988. Contains good info on how to write business plans, locate and raise capital, plan tax strategies, computerize—a book much like the one you're reading now, although written for small businesses in general.

Periodicals

- *SELF-EMPLOYED AMERICA, The News Publication For Your Small Business.* P.O. Box 612067, DFW Airport, TX 75261. Super publication for the truly small business person. There's a catch— you have to be a member of the National Association for the Self-Employed to receive this bi-monthly read. Drop a line to Karen C. Jones at the above address for particulars.
- *Women in Business.* The ABWA Co., 9100 Ward Parkway, Kansas City, MO 64114. Monthly column on business basics for women entrepreneurs and owners, plus other good stuff. Although aimed at women, most of us men could sneak a peek and gain a lot.

- *I.B.(Independent Business), America's Small Business Magazine.* F/S Publishing, Inc., #211, 875 S. Westlake Blvd., Westlake Village, CA 91361, (805) 496-6156. Top publication, covering tax tactics, small business computing, marketing moves, managing money, banking and finance, and business cost-savers—whatever is involved in running a small business.

TIME MANAGEMENT

Books

- Best, Fred. *Flexible Life Scheduling.* New York: Praeger Publishing, 1980. A scientific text. Only for those who want an in-depth and scholarly view of the study of time management. Not for the generalist. Takes an academic approach.
- Blanchard, Kenneth, and Spencer Johnson. *The One Minute Manager.* New York: William Morrow and Co., 1982. The single most influential book on time management ever written. This book, more than any other, awakened business people to the need to manage their time so they had time for life. Get it and read it! *Please.*
- Blanchard, Kenneth, William Oncken, Jr., and Hal Burrows. *The One Minute Manager Meets the Monkey.* New York: William Morrow and Co. 1989. The only better text might be the original *The One Minute Manager.* This is a must-read book that may literally save your professional life.
- Catlin, Steven A. *Work Less and Play More, How You Can Achieve the Leisure Life.* Santa Barbara, Calif.: Fithian Press, 1989. Enjoyable book with lots of good advice. Catlin gives a blueprint for an ulcer-free life and a plan for early retirement. Good read. Warning — this is a book that could change your life!
- Culp, Stephanie. *How to Get Organized When You Don't Have Time.* Cincinnati, Ohio: Writer's Digest Books, 1986. Fair to middling general text—covers the same ideas as most other books on the subject only in a less interesting way. Might be of value to those who want to know every single thought on the subject, but otherwise your time might be better spent in reading other sources.

- Davenport, Rita. *Making Time Making Money, A Step-by-Step Program to Set Your Goals and Achieve Success.* New York: St. Martin's Press, 1982. Fair to good text. Author takes a relatively simple concept and treats it as a complex one. Some worthwhile ideas, though.

Periodicals

- *Communication Briefings.* Encoders, Inc., Suite 110, 700 Black Horse Pike, Blackwood, NJ 08012. Good magazine on sound management techniques, including articles from time to time on effective time management.
- *Women in Business.* The ABWA Co., Inc., 9100 Ward Parkway, Kansas City, MO 64114. Excellent periodical for businesswomen and men. Various subjects of interest to the small business person, but they often publish good articles on time management as it relates to small business.
- *Executive Female.* NAFE, 127 W. 24th St., 4th Floor, New York, NY 10011. Several times a year will have good articles on time and stress management, along with other topical articles on business.

Articles

- Oncken, William. "Managing Management Time: Who's Got the Monkey?" Article in November 1974 issue of the *Harvard Business Review.* Generally acknowledged to be a classic—a timeless presentation of time management ills and how they can be cured. This article led to the book *The One Minute Manager Meets the Monkey.*

ET CETERA

- Edgerton, Leslie H. *You and Your Clients: Milady's Human Relations for Cosmetology.* Albany, NY:, Milady Publishing Co., 1992. Can be ordered from Milady Publishing Co. (A Division of Delmar Publishers, Inc.), 3 Columbia Circle, Box 12519, Albany, NY 12212-2519. A chance to blow my own horn! Seriously, this was my first book for Milady on the salon business, and I think you'll find it full of timely and valuable information on how to build a clientele list quickly. My original working title for *You and Your Clients* was "How to Bridge the Gap Between the Style Your Client *Has* . . . And the Style She *Wants*," and that is basically what the book is about—communication. Effective communication between stylist and client is the cornerstone of a successful salon, I feel, and in this text, I try to pass on twenty-five years of experience in this area. To be honest, I have stolen a lot of great ideas over the years from a lot of great stylists and salon owners, but say! . . . does that make me a bad person? As the kids say nowadays, "Not!" It just makes me a smart salon owner. Get it and steal some ideas for yourself!

INDEX